# HOW CHILDREN LEARN LANGUAGE

# HOW CHILDREN LEARN LANGUAGE

**James McLean, Ph.D.**
*Senior Scientist Emeritus*
*Bureau of Child Research*
*The University of Kansas*

**Lee K. McLean, Ph.D.**
*Professor of Educational Psychology*
*University of Connecticut*

SINGULAR PUBLISHING GROUP, INC.
SAN DIEGO · LONDON

**Singular Publishing Group, Inc.**
401 West "A" Street, Suite 325
San Diego, California 92101-7904

**Singular Publishing Ltd.**
19 Compton Terrace
London, N1 2UN, UK

**Singular Publishing Group, Inc.,** publishes textbooks, clinical manuals, clinical reference books, journals, videos, and multimedia materials on speech-language pathology, audiology, otorhinolaryngology, special education, early childhood, aging, occupational therapy, physical therapy, rehabilitation, counseling, mental health, and voice. For your convenience, our entire catalog can be accessed on our website at *http://www.singpub.com*. Our mission to provide you with materials to meet the daily challenges of the ever-changing health care/educational environment will remain on course if we are in touch with you. In that spirit, we welcome your feedback on our products. Please telephone (**1-800-521-8545**), fax (**1-800-774-8398**), or e-mail (*singpub@singpub.com*) your comments and requests to us.

Typeset in 11/13 Palatino by So Cal Graphics
Printed in the United States of America by McNaughton and Gunn

**Library of Congress Cataloging-in-Publication Data**

McLean, James E.
    How children learn language / James McLean, Lee K. McLean.
      p.  cm.
    Includes bibliographical references (p. ) and index.
    ISBN 1-56593-683-3 (pbk. : alk. paper)
      1. Language acquisition.  I. McLean, Lee K.  II. Title.
P118.M3934   1999
401'.93—dc21
                                     98-18592
                                          CIP

# CONTENTS

# PREFACE

A few years ago, Sadanand Singh, Chairman of Singular Publishing Group, remarked that one of the most frequent requests he received from educators at all levels of early childhood and special education was for a book about children's language development that was less technical than the standard textbooks. These professionals were not seeking to become scholars in developmental linguistics, but, because they were working directly with young children, they simply needed to better understand the nature, processes, and the dynamics of children's acquisition of this critically important human skill. Such knowledge would help them not only to support the language development of typically developing children, but also to better understand children with delays or serious disorders of language. It also would help them to participate more productively in any treatment programs being offered in their classrooms by professionals who were specialists in language development and its disorders.

Our aim in writing this book was to simply "tell the story" of the acquisition of communicative behaviors and language in a narrative that was accurate, but not so scholarly that it overwhelmed readers with every piece of research, detail, and every difference of perspective regarding the process. Citations are minimal and largely limited to the key researchers of the 1970s and 1980s who moved the field into today's predominant language theories. In addition, the book is organized to reflect our belief that communication and language development is not likely to be fully understood if one studies only the acquisition of linguistic skills. This is why we begin the "story" by describing the importance of children's social and physical environments, particularly the role of parents, in shaping the interactive context for teaching communicative and language skills. Following this, we present the baby's side of the story, so to speak, by describing how babies participate in the socialization process and the non-linguistic skills they must acquire to bring them to the point of developing language. With this information as a starting point, it is imminently clear why early language emerges as it does. It also gives an appreciation of the complexity of the process and how the process can go wrong.

We hope that instructors will find that the book is accurate in its presentation of the *gestalt* of the current theories about language development—even within its self-imposed limitations on technical comprehensiveness. Instructors should feel free to supplement any topic in the book with reports on current research and students should be encouraged to read more in-depth publications on any of the topics that pique their interest. Foremost, however, is our hope that professionals in nonlanguage fields will find this narrative to be comprehensible and interesting enough to meet their need to understand more about this miracle of a typical child's development of a socially functional language system in the first 3 years of life. And further, that such an understanding will help them to implement the rich communicative and language-learning environments needed by young children, including those with disabilities.

*To Dr. Richard Shiefelbusch whose Bureau of Child Research at the University of Kansas provided us with an academic home in which to acquire knowledge, and a rich professional work environment to do something with that knowledge*

# WHY CHILDREN LEARN TO TALK:

# THE ROLE OF LANGUAGE IN HUMAN SOCIETIES

## JAMES McLEAN

---

### Key Concepts

✔ Language exists as an efficient way for humans to communicate in a symbolic manner that is free from the constraints of space and time.

✔ Language is our primary means of survival and is, therefore, a critical human skill. It allows us to establish and maintain social compacts or cultures.

✔ Parents are naturally motivated to teach children to communicate and children are naturally suited to learn to communicate.

✔ Children must acquire special knowledge about people and things in their environment in order to acquire the communication and language skills of their culture.

---

## INTRODUCTION

When most people are asked to think about language, they usually think of a complex system of oral and written symbols, the combining of these symbols into words, and the rules for stringing these words together to form sentences. In other words, when people are asked to think of language, they usually think first of its *linguistic structure*. Clearly, languages have complex structures and they have complex rules. When most people think of language, however, they do *not* often think about why it exists and where humans would be if it did not exist. Yet, these questions about the *reasons* for language figure prominently in gaining an understanding of children's ability and motivation to learn the language of their culture.

Similarly, when most people are asked to think about *how* children learn language, they most often think of their first words, phrases, and sentences. Again, our first instinct is to think about the linguistic structure of language that is acquired by young children. As they try to go beyond the structure of children's early language, most people find that they have little idea about exactly how children learn this structure They intuitively know that children learn language from what they hear from parents, siblings, other family members, and playmates. They also know that there is a gradual process for language development but are frequently stumped when they try to explain the details and the dynamics of this process. Most of all, however, most people do not realize what children must know *before* they are able to acquire language. Yet, it is this understanding of the huge body of knowledge that children bring to the language learning process that makes that learning process more logical and, thus, more understandable to professionals who are not experts in child language development.

In this first chapter, then, we will discuss why language exists. We will offer a broad look at how language is taught by others. We will also discuss how language is used and why it is so critical to the human condition. We will also take an overview look at the kinds of knowledge children must have in order to acquire first communication and then language.

By offering these initial, broad views of the nature of language, we hope to set the stage for the content of the remaining chapters in this book. If readers are to truly understand how and why children learn language, they must resensitize themselves to the nature of language that is beyond its structure. They must appreciate the body of nonlanguage knowledge that children must acquire to make the learning of their language possible. They must also recognize the nature of the strategies and efforts that the people around children apply to help them in the process of first learning to *communicate* and then learning the language structures needed to expand and extend their communicative abilities to the levels needed to perform successfully in the culture in which they live. In other words, language learning is not just about learning language structure. It is about learning to live in a social world of other people and the relationships between and among these people. It is also about learning to live in a physical world of millions of entities and relationships between and among those entities. Each of the first four chapters of this book focuses on a piece of this overall process by which children gather the formidable body knowledge about their physical and social world. For it is this body of knowledge that undergirds the learning and the use of language itself.

This approach is the "long way around" to understanding children's acquisition of language. But is the sure way and the most logical way. In this overall exposition, the reader will encounter much about child development that he or she already knows. But by reviewing the elements of this existing knowledge about early child development and connecting it with the specific elements of learning communication and language, readers will be able to see the logic and the sense of the overall process.

Between 12 and 18 months of age, typically developing babies utter their first *word*. By 36 months of age the same children have a vocabulary of over a thousand words that they can combine in phrases and sentences up to seven or eight words long. At 36 months they can make statements and ask questions. They can request things—politely. They can talk about future events and recount experiences that they have had in the past. They can "promise." They can give orders. They can tell lies. In the space of the 24 months, between their first birthday and their third, most typically developing children have mastered the basic elements of human speech and their culture's spoken language. From 3 years of age on, it is but a matter of increasing their vocabulary, refining their grammar, and increasing their abilities to use their language more effectively and efficiently.

This rapid process of language development by young children is something that we tend to take for granted. In fact, however, it is a process that babies work very hard at. It is also a process to which parents, preschool teachers, and other significant adults and children in a baby's environment contribute considerable attention and effort. Yet, despite all that we do to help our babies acquire communication and language skills, most of us have only vague notions about how our children learn these two important skills. Beyond some awareness that we have talked to our babies, helped them to say several hundred words and phrases, and responded to many thousands of their utterances over the years, most of us don't quite understand how systematically and predictably we have behaved in order to help our children master their language. If we don't fully understand what it is that we, as teaching adults, have done, it is certain that most of us don't fully understand what the children have done either.

It is truly amazing that children can acquire a basic competence in one of the most complex of human behaviors during the 3 years that begin at birth and end about the time that they move out of the toddler stage. How do they do it?

The most general answer to this question has two parts. First, typically developing infants have intact human brains that are uniquely capable of learning the language system used in their culture. The concept and details of spoken and written languages were developed by human brains thousands of years ago. Language, then, is a very complex and important human behavioral system whose elements and mechanics have been designed *by* and *for* the specific abilities of the *human brain*.

Second to the brain's ability to acquire language are parents and other people in children's social environments who play crucial and effective roles in children's language development process. Adults in every human culture create a special caregiving and teaching environment for their young children. This environment is structured both to insist that children learn their culture's language and, then, to help them to do it. Although the adults in a child's environment do not sit down and consciously and formally teach their culture's language to children, it is true that language is *taught* to young children by the adults and other children around them who already know it. Moreover, it is taught in ways that leave no doubt that it is considered one of the most important things in the world for a child to learn. On the other side of the partnership, young children are mentally equipped and highly motivated to learn this critical human skill.

## UNDERSTANDING LANGUAGE DEVELOPMENT

In this book, we will talk about how language is taught to, and learned by, children. We will emphasize how universal this process is. Most people instinctively know how to teach language to young children. After all, millions of parents have taught children to talk perfectly well without studying language acquisition in college. The problem is that most parents and other adults are not consciously aware of their own knowledge about their language system, nor about how they teach language to children. Even parents who have helped several of their own children learn to talk often cannot describe the process or explain their role in it. Therefore, one of the things that we will try to do in this book is to make you more aware of how much you already instinctively know about language and about how it is taught to and learned by young children. As a consequence, one of the more important abilities that you should get from reading this book is how to talk about children's language development and the role that parents, and other significant people in a child's environment, have in the process. It is not until we are able to *talk* about our knowledge that we truly understand what we know. Thus the organization of our knowledge and the learning of the vocabulary needed to talk about language development will strengthen and clarify our knowledge about it.

Serious problems in speech and language development have major, negative consequences for children. As a consequence, educators and other professionals and paraprofessionals who work with young children or with children with disabilities need to know more about both the processes and the products of children's speech and language development. This book is an attempt to guide their mastery of that knowledge. When these important professionals better understand *why* and *how* children learn language, and *what* it is that they learn as they progress from those first crude attempts at words at 1 year of age to thousands of well-structured sentences at 3 years of age, they will be better prepared to deal with children who have serious problems in the areas of speech and language. They also will be better prepared to call for, and support, the special efforts needed to help children better their skills in these crucial behavioral domains.

Because language is a complex system, most people assume that understanding its development must be an extremely complex task. This is simply not true. A professional in education, child care, or health care does not need to know all of the technical details of a language's three-level linguistic system or all of the intricacies of its acquisition processes to have a good understanding of the early language development process. There are specialists in speech-language pathology, psycholinguistics, and child development who can explain and apply the more technical aspects of this process when and if such information is needed. However, there is much that one can know about the why and how of language learning that does not require being a specialist. Having a broad and basic knowledge about the language learning process will allow you to understand where a child is in his or her language development, why he or she might be at this stage, and what help might be necessary to help him or her progress to higher stages. Today, we recognize that children who are at risk for failure because of either extreme economic disadvantage or mental or physical disabilities will benefit more from *inclusion* in typical day-care, early education, or special school settings with their age peers. However, children with special needs who are included in mainstream settings must have the support of parents, educators, and care providers who understand their special needs.

As a result of our cultural commitment to children with special needs, more and more educators in Head Start, early childhood education, and special education are coming face-to-face with children who may not be developing an appropriate or adequate language system. Thus, having basic knowledge and insights into the process and the products of children's language development will enable professionals who are not specialists in language development to not only improve the speech and language teaching in their own environments, but also prepare them to interact more effectively with professionals who provide specialized therapy services to children with speech and language problems. Such knowledgeable professionals will also be more effective and sensitive in dealing with children who have speech and language delays, and, as importantly, with their families.

In addition to increased professional competence, professionals in education can also have the satisfaction and the pleasure of understanding and fully appreciating this exciting process as they observe and help children in their own families. At some time, most extended families have concerns about the language development of one or more of their children. Thus, this knowledge can create additional sources for information and direction within these families.

**What we hope to accomplish in this book, then, is to provide you with the *sense* of the speech and language development process, because it is an eminently *sensible* process.**

Besides being a sensible process, language learning is also a universal human process that one can readily understand with a bit of guided study. Beginning to understand the language development process requires that we first reawaken our appreciation of what it takes to create and maintain a human society and what it takes to live successfully in one.

Many accounts of language development begin with the study of what language *is* and quickly move into the complexity of a language system's elements with its three levels of structure:

Speech sounds (phonology),

Meaning units (morphology), and

Rules for stringing them together (syntax).

Our approach to teaching the logic and "sense" of language development, however, will not begin with the structural elements of language systems as identified in descriptive linguistics. Instead, we will emphasize what language *does* for people and their societies. This understanding of what language does, and how it does it, sets the stage for a sensible and deeper understanding of why and how young children learn language. This aspect of language is referred to as the *pragmatics* of language—its practical uses among humans.

## WHAT LANGUAGE DOES IN HUMAN SOCIETIES

Imagine yourself at lunch in a small restaurant in which you can hear the conversations at several of the tables in the room. What would you hear?

"So I said to my wife—it's a good buy. Why don't we go for it? So we did. What do you think?"

"I think it was a good buy, too. Where did you say you found it for that price?"

"Bobby's teacher said that he must be better prepared when he comes to class. In other words—more homework."

"Do you think you can get him to study better at home? Do you have the same type of computer that he uses at school?"

"Do you think that you could pick me up in the morning? Bill needs the car to go to Kansas City."

"Gee, Gwen, tomorrow's a bad day for me to take our car, too—I'll call Grace and see if she can pick both of us up, Okay?"

"What are you going to order?"

"I'm thinking about a good greasy cheeseburger—how about you?"

"Unfortunately, that *does* sound good. My doctor will hate me."

"Well, that's my idea, what do you think?"

"I think that you're looking at the problem from the wrong angle. Do you want to know what I'd do?"

"Yes. You're better at these things than I am."

"I'd sure love to have another iced tea.

"Another tea? I'll see if I can catch the waiter's eye."

"I'm sorry—I've got to run, I've got to pick up the kids and get them to soccer practice. Can you meet me for lunch Thursday—maybe a little earlier?"

"I understand, go on. Thursday's fine, I'll look forward to it."

These conversations are ordinary—just what you would hear anywhere, anytime. You are hearing our culture's language at work. What does it do? One common response to this question is, "Well, language allows people to express their thoughts and their ideas." That's true enough, but there is more. Why are people expressing their thoughts and ideas? In these examples, people are using their language ability to *conduct the business of living in a human social environment.*

The important thing to realize here is that the daily business of interacting productively with other people in our society or culture means that we use language to *have effects on other people.* These effects can vary widely. Perhaps a speaker is seeking another person's reassurance about an idea. Perhaps he or she is requesting help in some way—perhaps to work together towards some common goal or task. Maybe a speaker is seeking approval, attention, sympathy, or perhaps he or she simply wants information. Whatever a speaker's immediate goal, his or her language is formulated and directed to evoke the desired response or action from another person or persons. Whatever effect a speaker hopes to have on another person, it is clear that the act of producing a language utterance is, at its most basic level, an *act* on another person. It is an act that anticipates that the receiver of the utterance will respond, hopefully in the way the speaker desires.

What does it mean to say that a language utterance is an act on another person? Since this is not an everyday awareness for most of us, it might serve us better to approach this notion from a broader perspective. To better grasp this concept, it helps to recognize that each of us lives in a complex world of thousands of people and thousands of things. To survive and thrive in that world, we must learn how to make our people world work in ways that provide us with the kinds of events and results that we desire from it. Thus, we must develop a set of appropriate and effective skills for operating on, and with, the *people* in their environment. It is these skills that provide entry into a cooperative, constructive human society. We are social animals, and we have built our many different world cultures on our abilities to work, play, and learn from one another. From day one, infants begin learning the basic skills needed to operate in the world of people. It is from the application of these skills that they acquire the vast body of knowledge and special abilities needed to live successfully and productively in both their social and physical environments.

As we saw earlier in the samples of everyday conversation, we need many things from other people. We need their attention and approval. We need their help in all of the domains that make up the day-to-day world of work, play, and learning. We need their knowledge and viewpoints on everything from politics to books and movies and the human condition. How can we act on people to make them respond to us in these ways? We can use certain physical acts on them, and we do. We sometimes use tugs, pushes, hugs, and other motor acts on them. However, such acts are extremely limited in both their level of societal acceptability and their range of usefulness. There are other types of motor acts that we can use to affect people. We can, for example, make gestures with our hands and our bodies or make faces that connote surprise, pain, pleasure, or displeasure. But these gestural and facial expressions are also limited in their usefulness. Such acts are often so ambiguous that others can only guess at the specific response we desire from them. Although these gestural, facial, and body acts can be useful at certain times and in certain circumstances, it is easy to see that much of what we want from other people requires more than we can accomplish with motor acts alone. This is why languages were developed by our ancestors. By producing certain words and phrases out of the millions that we are capable of, it is possible for us to *act* on other people in rather precise and efficient ways—ways that will have an extremely high probability of achieving the specific responses that we desire from them. In this sense, then, the rich collection of language acts that we learn to produce constitutes the keystone of our social behavior.

## THE BASIC RULES THAT ALLOW LANGUAGE ACTS TO WORK ON OTHER PEOPLE

Let's return briefly to our examples of restaurant conversations. If you had observed the participants in the conversations as they were played out, you would have noticed that the people seated around the table were generally attending to whomever was speaking and listening carefully to what he or she was saying. Some of these partners might have nodded at the speaker or reacted to the message with a frown or a smile. All, or at least most, of the listeners prepared and produced some conversational *response* to a speaker's question or statement. After producing an utterance, the previous *speaker* turned into a *receiver* and was equally attentive and responsive to the new speaker.

This pattern of mutual responsiveness and exchange of speaker-listener roles, reveals the commitments that we, as social beings, make to one another in our language exchanges. These commitments are actually "rules" that we all follow as we interact conversationally with other people in our society. These rules have been described by language philosophers (Gordon & Lakoff, 1975; Grice 1975) who noted that, first of all, we follow a rule that says, "We will listen to what another person is saying." After listening we will further commit ourselves to making a sincere effort to understand, exactly, what message the other person *intends* for us to receive. Even further, we are committed to make a sincere and polite effort to respond cooperatively and constructively to that message.

At this point in our discussion, we have emphasized the fact that language is our primary *means* for conducting the business of living in a society with other people who use our language. The fact that language is so vital for making the social aspects of our environment work explains why the members of a culture who already know the language work so diligently to teach their young children how to use it appropriately and effectively. The rules for our use of language show clearly that a society is *committed to making language work.* As members of that society, we attend to what is being said to us. We do our best to understand the intentions of the person speaking to us, and we make every effort to make sure that what a speaker says, works for him or her. If we cannot respond in the way that we think a conversational partner wants us to, then we most often will try to help him or her to arrive at a statement, question, or request that we can respond to constructively. Let us show you a few examples of how we do this in everyday conversations.

"I just hate that man. I think he's dishonest and despicable, don't you?"

"Well, I wouldn't say that."

"You're right, perhaps that is too strong. Would you agree that he needs to be treated with some caution when one negotiates a deal with him?"

"I guess I'd agree with that; but I think that's a good rule when negotiating with anyone."

"Mommy, I want some cookies."

"Okay, but you can only have one otherwise you won't want any dinner later."

"But, I'm real hungry—can't I have three?"

"Well, let's go with just two cookies, okay?" (Gives two cookies)

"Okay, two."

"What do you say?"

"Thank-you."

"You're welcome. But you had better eat a good dinner."

In a conversation, both the speaker and the receiver general-ly make it clear that, as social beings, they are committed to a *co-operative, constructive,* and *polite* partnership with our fellows. These commitments are the cornerstone of human societies; and our use of language according to strict rules is one of the most obvious expressions of these commitments.

## A MORE BASIC LOOK AT WHY
## HUMAN SOCIETIES NEED LANGUAGE

As a final point in our attempt to establish a broader perspective on why we need to be able to *act* on other people with language, we should consider the fact that the human animal is among the least well-equipped to survive in a hostile universe on physical prowess alone. We are slow when compared to other species. Our claws are woeful. Our fangs are relatively ineffective against everything but a tender *filet mignon.*

Clearly then, humans have survived on earth because of their ability to band together in social compacts or tribes in which the considerable labor of living can be divided among many. Further, we have survived because each advance in our abilities to achieve certain important goals could be made available to all of the members of our immediate tribe through our language sys-tem. Even more importantly, we have survived because each *gen-eration's* knowledge and skills in designing and building the many tools, weapons, and products that human societies need have been transmitted across time and space to succeeding gen-erations. Consequently, each succeeding human generation is able to begin at the highest level of knowledge and ability at-tained by the generations that preceded it.

This transmission of skills and knowledge across time and space is perhaps the most profound function of human language and we need not go back to the discovery of fire and the wheel to appreciate that fact. We need only to look at a classroom of children being instructed in the discoveries of the past to realize that in our current culture, approximately the first 21 years of a human's life are spent learning the already established skills and knowledge needed to survive in a modern world which is, essentially, people-made.

It is at this point that we can resensitize ourselves to the realization that our language is our *primary means of survival*, perhaps more so now than when it was used to organize a hunt for food animals, pass on knowledge about how to plant and harvest, make a spear or wheel, or build a fire. It requires vast amounts of both broad and specific knowledge to live in a modern society. In today's world, the production and services labor needed to maintain a society are so specialized and extensive that they must be shared by all of the individuals in that society. As a result of this division of labor among all of us, an individual member rarely participates in the full chain of production for any one of the thousands of things needed by a modern society. For example, only a small segment of our society is involved in the direct growing of food. However, many thousands of other people are involved in industries that process and prepare foodstuffs. More thousands are involved in the logistics by which the foodstuffs are delivered across vast distances. Still others are involved in the grocery business, which manages the distribution of these foodstuffs to millions of people through the use of a monetary system that, itself, depends on thousands of other people-run industries, such as banks and other financial institutions. Clearly, each of these specialized segments of a modern society requires intensive organization, coordination, and knowledge to fulfill its role in the thousands of production chains that maintain that society. These production chains produce everything in our society from food and clothing to work tools and defense armaments. They provide education to the full range of our society. They produce the tools of our leisure, such as books, movies, and music. Thus, our modern societies require that people work together cooperatively for the common good of all. Each of us must be able to coordinate a significant portion of our thoughts and actions in ways that are complementary to one another and, thus, contribute to the goals we have set for our particular segment of society. Modern societies with their wide ranging needs and complex institutions simply would not be possible without language.

We should note here that it is possible to coordinate some relatively cooperative social scenarios without language. For example, we might use pointing or extended-palm "request" gestures to communicate with others. We sometimes do this in noisy environments or when someone is across the room. However, if we could only act on others using gestures, we would quickly find serious limitations to accomplishing anything very complex. With such gestures, for example, one can only indicate things that are present in the context of the interaction. So, using only gestures, how would you ask for something that is not present in the immediate environment or communicate about something you did yesterday or perhaps 2 months ago? Without a complex, symbolic language system it would be next to impossible to develop and maintain the human societies needed to maintain our species on the earth.

Indeed, each individual culture or element of a society not only requires a unifying full language system, but it also requires hundreds of specialized, secondary languages that are designed for specialized communicative needs. Most farmers in America speak English—but they also use many words and phrases that are not in the vocabulary of many people who live in cities. The financial workers of our societies have a specialized, secondary language, as do engineers, physicists, physicians, teachers, and hundreds of other segments our society that have specialized training or specialized roles. As we will discuss in a later chapter, each member of a society has several sublanguages that he or she uses in everyday life. Most people use a slightly different language at work than they use at home or with old friends or with new acquaintances. These sublanguages include different vocabularies as well as differing levels of politeness and formality. Men often use a sublanguage language that is different from one that a woman might use. Indeed, the more specialized sublanguages that a person has, the better prepared he or she is to succeed in his or her socialized world of other people. Can you remember hearing such admonitions as:

"You're using a lot of jargon that I don't understand. Can you

say that in plain English?"

"Don't you ever talk that way to your mother again."

"I don't appreciate your tone of voice."

"Well, **lah**-di-dah! Aren't you getting fancy."

Those comments were intended by others to teach you when *not* to use a certain one of your many sublanguages! We will talk more about this later, when we look at what parents and other adults do and say when they are helping children to learn their language.

## So, Why Do Children Learn to Talk and Why Do Parents and Others Work So Diligently to Help Them?

With the realization that language is critical to the creation and maintenance of human societies, the underlying motivations for the learning and teaching of language skills are obvious. But few of us think consciously about these more profound aspects of human language use when we begin our efforts to teach our children to talk. Rather, we are instinctively following the lessons of our ancestors when we begin to teach our children about their specific culture's language system.

It is both important and compelling to every human society to teach children to talk. As members of a society, we want to make it possible for a child to conduct his or her social business. We want children to be able to do the things with language that we listed in the first paragraphs of this chapter. We want them to be able to ask for things—politely. We want them to be able to ask questions. We also want them to be able to "promise" and to make comments about things they like—or don't like. We want them able to acquire all of the knowledge from the past that will be important in their lives. We want them to be able to exchange views and knowledge with other children so that they can understand the world from other people's perspectives and learn that their own views are not always universally accepted.

We want our children to be able to do these things because we know these are the things one must do to "belong" and to function successfully in a world of people. If one cannot use a language effectively with other people, one cannot build the many cooperative relationships that are required to live in a society.

You know, for example, that most people in this country who are deaf learn American Sign Language. You may also be aware that many deaf people consider themselves to have a unique culture because of their unique language. Many people with deafness have also learned to produce spoken language. Among the deaf who can use speech, however, only those who can *also* use their culture's manual sign language are accepted as being full members of the "true" *deaf culture* by many persons who are deaf. A related example is the legislation in France that insists that the French language must be protected from the intrusion of American words so as to preserve the *true* French culture. All of these examples serve to emphasize the role of language in establishing and maintaining human social compacts or cultures.

To be a language user, then, is to be a fully functioning member of one of the thousands of different human societies. If one is able to speak several languages, he or she can literally function in, and belong to, several cultures. Language is, in a sense, the *essence* of the socialization of *Homo sapiens*. It is the basis for both survival and for excelling in a society. It is, then, a critical skill to be taught to our offspring.

## How Best Can We Come to Understand the Process of Language Acquistion?

In this book we emphasize the teaching and learning of a culture's language as an *interactive* process that involves the people in a culture who can already produce the language and new members of that culture who cannot yet do so. It is an orderly process.

- It is a process that begins early in a baby's life.

- It is a process that requires the child to acquire many different kinds of knowledge, much of it learned long before a baby is ready to produce speech or language.

- It is a process that requires a coordination of the efforts of both the teacher and the learner.

- It is a process that changes throughout its course, with both teachers and learners adapting and fine-tuning their efforts to match and fully benefit from the behaviors of the others involved.

If we are to understand the full process of language learning we must take detailed looks at the full range of early, *nonlanguage*, developmental processes that parallel and undergird the development of language. Each of these distinct, but related, processes is directed toward young children's acquisition of certain bodies of knowledge and certain behavioral skills. Each different body of knowledge and repertoire of behavior that children acquire contributes in separate, but specific, ways to the overall developmental process that all typical children move through. At the end of these earliest developmental processes, we find typically developing children who can interact cooperatively with other people, work and play effectively among the elements of their physical environment, and use their language in appropriate and relatively efficient ways.

Obviously, it takes a lot of teaching and a lot of learning for a child to reach this state of relative effectiveness as a member of a human society. Clearly, to describe these several teaching and learning processes, we as authors, must have a plan for doing so. In developing the plan for this book, we acted with the overriding belief that one cannot understand the acquisition of language by looking at only the acquisition of the linguistic forms that make up human language. Rather, one must look at all of the elements that come *before* a child begins to talk. It is only when one looks at the kinds of experiences and knowledge a child gains throughout the early developmental period and *brings to* the language learning process that he or she can understand *how* the child can learn language and *why* the child learns the language elements that he or she learns. Thus, we now need to take a brief first look at the nature and the products of this early developmental process.

## THE ELEMENTS OF THE EARLY DEVELOPMENTAL PROCESS

The first 3 years of the typical human infant's life offer an amazingly rich and complex body of experiences that result in an equally amazing complex body of infant development and learning. This early developmental period sees the child develop rapidly and orderly along two broad fronts: physical and mental.

## Physical Development

In the first 3 years of life babies grow from around 1 foot to about 3 feet long. Their weight increases in proportion to their growth in length. Their motor abilities move from a state of practical helplessness to a point where they can crawl and, finally, walk and run. At the end of this early period of development, they can typically use their arms and hands to perform increasingly skilled motor acts, including the relatively refined manipulation of objects and the ability to throw and, sometimes, even catch them. In the first 3 years, then, children physically metamorphize from small and helpless infants into small people who can manage themselves in their overall environment with amazing skill and energy. All of these changes occur as cells divide and grow, brains and neural systems grow and stabilize, and motor movements come under predictable, and more precise, neurological control.

## Mental (Cognitive) Development

Just as physical development has many dimensions, mental development also occurs along several separate, but related, fronts. Children's mental development is referred to as their *cognitive* development; and this developmental continuum stretches across a complex of learning domains that reflect the complexity of the human social and physical environments that children must learn to master. These cognitive learning domains include social development, sensorimotor development, and symbolic development. They also include the precursors of higher level cognitive abilities, such as reasoning and other conceptual skills. The acme of cognitive development in early childhood is the acquisition of nonlinguistic communicative acts and, then, the language system of their home culture. Although progress along the many domains of children's learning involves different natures and processes, they also interact with each other. These interactions between and among the many learning domains involved in early cognitive development are critical. It is the summing and integration of all of these separate domains that produces children's overall cognitive abilities to function successfully and productively in an environment that demands their eventual broad repertoire of social, motor, and conceptual skills.

The very complexity of all of these cognitive developmental domains, along with their many critical interactions and integrations, makes a simple exposition on them impossible. An organizational dichotomy suggested by renowned developmental psychologist Jerome Bruner (1973) is most helpful in gaining an understanding of the many dimensions of the general cognitive domain developing in these early years of life. Bruner suggested that the earliest elements of cognitive development can be productively organized along two lines:

1. " People Skills" and

2. "Thing Skills."

Each of these broad headings covers many separate skills and we will be discussing these in some detail throughout this book. At this point, however, we want to give you a broad perspective on these two categories of skill domains.

## People Skills

In this chapter, we have emphasized that ours is a social world in which we are dependent on one another for our well being. Compared to other mammal species, humans take a long time to mature and prepare themselves for a long and productive life. This process begins as babies are made a part of their social world by helping them learn that other people are sources of comfort, help, information, and pleasure. The process continues as we help our babies learn how to belong to, and function successfully in, that world of other people. Children must learn many things to become successful in the world of people and the eventual acquisition of language is the key to most of them. However, babies must learn many things about their world of people before they are able to master language. We will track the development of people skills in very young children beginning with their learning the rudiments of how to interact effectively with other people, how to affect the behaviors of others, and, finally, how to use language to meet the expectations and requirements of full membership in their culture.

## Thing Skills

Just as babies must learn about their social world and how best to use it, they must also learn about the physical things that surround them. In the same sense that they must learn certain skills to operate in their social world, they must also acquire the skills to function productively in their physical world of things. They must learn to hold and manipulate things. They must learn how to act on things to achieve their desired results. They must learn the relationships that obtain between and among things. They must learn, for example, that some things go into other things and that some objects must be used to make another object perform in a certain way. In many ways, babies must acquire a basic knowledge of the world of *physics.*

In addition, children must acquire a sense of the kinds of objects that surround them. They must catalog these entities in terms of their purposes, their uses, and even their ownership—is it *mine* or *mommy's*? They must learn that, when a thing disappears from their immediate environment, it still exists in another location. There is much work to be done to help children discover and learn about their physical world of things.

## People and Thing Skills as a Requirement for Language

If you think about it, you can readily see that both people and things must be in place before true language is possible. The language we use *refers* to the people and things in our environment. A key program of research in the 1970s by Lois Bloom (Bloom, 1970, 1973) provided the data that sensitized us to the most basic fact about our use of language—we *talk* about what we *know*. Thus, babies can only talk about (refer to) what they already know about. And, as we will see throughout this book, babies' primary reason for talking is to have effects on the people around them. By the time they acquire a language, babies know a great deal about other people and the rules for how and why to have the effects on them that they desire to have. These facts are the bases for our position that, if people are to truly understand how and why children learn a language, they must understand all the teaching and learning that occurs *before* language emerges as well as the process that is focused on the acquisition of language itself.

## THE PLAN OF STUDY

Breaking down the elements of the many teaching and learnng processes that result in language is a challenge. We will begin our more detailed study of the overall process by looking at the role that parents and other significant adults in a child's life play in it. Thus, in Chapter 2, we will look at all of the ways that adults arrange children's social and physical environments to guide and help children achieve all of the different learning goals that are involved in both the basic *socialization* of very young children and the attainment of the early, and most basic, *cognitive* abilities that they acquire in their first year of development.

At about the end of their first year of life, children's learning includes many abilities and skills that signal parents that they are ready to begin to acquire the *linguistic system* that makes up their environment's spoken language. In Chapter 3, therefore, we will look at the strategies and actions of parents and other adults and older children as they focus more specifically on helping children acquire this complex and demanding system.

In Chapter 4, we will take an equally detailed look at what children contribute to this process of acquiring the knowledge and skills necessary to use the language of their culture. Children actively work at learning, and they demonstrate specific strategies that help them in their acquisition of the early sensorimotor, social, and nonverbal communication skills that will be important in the eventual learning of their full language system. The acquisition of this early knowledge base requires the best, most effective efforts of both the teacher and the learner to succeed. Children also display some very effective strategies for learning first to comprehend and then to produce, their culture's spoken language. By understanding the strategies that children apply in this overall process, adults will better understand what they need to do in their various roles with children.

In Chapter 5, we will review and summarize the development of the several of the specific *nonlinguistic* skills that young children acquire. These varying skills and knowledge holdings are most crucial in the development of children's ability to learn and use their native language, as well as to master their complex physical environment. Therefore, we want these knowledge holdings to be fresh in the reader's mind as we move on to the learning of language itself. The most important of these nonlinguistic skills include the learning of both "thing skills" and "people skills." Among the more advanced people skills examined in this chapter are those that are communicative in that they are intended to have effects on people—but are not specifically linguistic.

In Chapter 6, we are finally ready to look at the specifics of *linguistic learning* itself. At that point in our study, we will have a good understanding that, at the point that children begin to talk, they have a vast knowledge base about both their social and physical world. By the time you get to this chapter, you will already know the details of that knowledge base and we will look at how this knowledge guides and shapes a child's learning and use of language elements and structures.

Finally, in Chapter 7, we will look at the breakdowns and problems that can occur in the speech-language development process and we will talk about the major causes of such breakdowns. We will examine the effects of certain childhood disabilities and environmental factors and how these can interact to cause problems in the language learning process. We will also identify the "red flags" that can alert a parent, caregiver, or professional that a child may be falling behind in his or her language development and what should be done when a language delay is suspected. Finally, we will offer suggestions for designing environments that will support young children's language development.

## SUMMARY

- Language plays a crucial role in the creation and maintenance of human societies. It allows us to band together in coordinated and cooperative groups in which each member is committed to interact with the other members of the group.

- Language allows us to construct complex and mutually serving social compacts and relationships for work and play.

- Language and socialization allow us to share our acquired knowledge and past experiences with others in the present and across future time lines.

- The human brain is uniquely designed to create, teach, learn, and use language.

- All human socieites share a strong drive to see that their offspring acquire the ability to learn and use language as soon as it is possible for them to do so.

- As infants and toddlers develop, they acquire "people skills" and "thing skills" from the social and physical environment in which they live. These skills lay the foundation for the acquisition of communication and language.

## References

Bloom, L. (1970). *Language development: Form and function in emerging grammars.* Cambridge, MA: M.I.T. Press.

Bloom, L. (1973). *One word at a time: The use of single word utterances before syntax.* The Hague, The Netherlands: Mouton.

Bruner, J. (1973). Organisation of early skills action. *Child Development,* *44,* 1–11.

Gordon, D., & Lakoff, G. (1975). Conversational postulates. In P. Cole & J. L. Morgan (Eds.), *Syntax and semantics: 3: Speech acts* (pp. 83–106). New York: Academic Press.

Grice, H. P. (1975). Logic and conversation. In P. Cole & J. L. Morgan (Eds.), *Syntax and semantics: 3. Speech acts* (pp. 41–58). New York: Academic Press.

# 2

# THE ROLE OF PARENTS AND OTHER ADULTS IN THE EARLY SOCIALIZATION AND COGNITIVE DEVELOPMENT OF VERY YOUNG CHILDREN

## JAMES McLEAN

---

## Key Concepts

✔ Parents and other people in babies' environments *make* them communicators before they understand communication by assigning communicative meaning to babies' nonverbal actions or states.

✔ Parents, caregivers, and siblings naturally adjust the way they talk to babies to be responsive to their needs and interact with them. They also talk about what is most meaningful to babies: the here and now.

✔ Language is learned against the backdrop of human interaction beginning with two basic behaviors: joint attention and turn taking.

---

✔ As parents begin to use words to affect their babies' behavior, babies come to understand that words are acts on other people and that other people will respond to those words.

✔ Babies progress from being passive communicators—parents and others assign meaning to their behaviors—to being active communicators by producing *nonlanguage* behaviors, such as body language and gestures, that are intended to evoke responses from the people around them.

# INTRODUCTION

The human infant enters the world virtually helpless. In the ensuing 3 years, the typical infant will become a relatively competent social partner, will learn much about the physical world in which he or she lives, and will know the rudiments of the language of the culture into which he or she was born. In addition to innate instincts, the newborn infant requires a well-designed set of environmental experiences through which he or she can discover and acquire the wide range of knowledge and skills needed to survive and prosper in his or her new environment. The knowledge and skills babies must acquire will come to the them from the environment into which they are born. That is, babies' learning is fueled by their direct experiences with the people and things of their environment . We looked briefly at the knowledge and skills that children must acquire early in life, and we know that much of this learning must occur *before* they can acquire language. In this chapter we will explore the role that parents (and other people in the children's environment) play in facilitating this learning.

We will begin by looking at the early socialization of children; that is, how they are brought into the world of other people—people who will then guide and teach them how to interact appropriately and productively with them. These early, but critical, learning experiences are most often provided by parents, although other adults and older children in the environment also contribute to the process. The early learning that we will discuss in this chapter includes the development of social interactions, adults' early use of language to children, and children's development of nonlinguistic communicative behaviors.

In Chapter 3, we will look at the activities of people in children's environment as they move on to the teaching of language itself. For now, however, we will concentrate on how children are *prepared* to learn language.


## BRINGING NEWBORNS INTO THE WORLD OF PEOPLE AND THINGS

Because the abilities to use and understand language are so basic to life in any culture, its members must be sure that their children acquire these abilities. However, language does not spring magically from the minds of children. Instead, among many other things, children must be helped to learn what language is and what it does. Then, they must learn to produce it and use it in the ways other members of the culture insist that it be used. The design and management of children's experiences in ways that facilitate the language learning process is, basically, *teaching*; and the teaching of language to its children is one of the primary goals of every human culture. However, we know that acquisition of language requires that children have a wide range of knowledge that is not specific to language. Thus the adults and other people in children's environment begin the process of preparing them for language learning by first helping babies to experience and appreciate the pleasure, knowledge, and security that emanate from their social world. Preparation for learning language begins immediately after the birth of a child. Actually, in some real ways, it probably begins *before* a child's birth.


### Early Preparation for Socialization and Language: Mother's Talk to Preborns and Newborns

Is there a mother in our Western culture who didn't start talking to her baby while she was carrying it? Perhaps, but is more likely that she began "conversations" with her baby early in her pregnancy.

"Oh my, we're a little restless today. I can feel you moving around. Ouch, quit kicking me!"

"Oh, did that noise scare you? It's all right, it was just your brother playing with his blocks. He is a little noisy isn't he? I'll see if I can calm him down."

"Oh, my back hurts. Will you hurry up and be born?"

"Let's get our bath and get dressed shall we? Daddy's taking us out to dinner. Won't that be nice?"

Conversations like these are called rhetorical because it is clear that there will be no answers or other spoken responses to the statements and questions that mothers offer to their yet un-born babies. It is interesting to note, however, that the intonations and inflections of a mother's utterances are very much like those used in a regular conversation in which a response is expected from a conversational partner. However, mothers in these pre-birth scenarios will probably talk just a bit louder than normal and they will also talk a bit more slowly. Typically, mothers will use complete sentences, repeat a lot, and exaggerate their normal inflections a bit so that the tonal patterns of their speech are more melodic and easy to hear. Often, then, mothers' speech to their unborn babies (and newborns as well) sounds rather "sing-songy." These patterns are so prevalent in Western cultures that they are readily recognized. Experts in language use a special name for these language and speech patterns used by mothers with preborns and very young children. They refer to them as "motherese" or "parentese."

There are several other characteristics of mothers' talk to their babies. For example, parentese is rarely angry in tone; in fact, it is most often "sweet-talk." In these one-way "conversa-tions," mothers are instinctively *beginning* to teach their children that spoken language is a good thing. Although it is impossible to say how much unborn children might actually be learning from these "conversations" with their mothers, we do know that they are being strongly conditioned to human speech and lan-guage and, thus, are becoming comfortable with its sounds, rhythms, and patterns through countless hours of experiencing their mothers' utterances. There is research that indicates that very young babies readily discriminate between "happy" and "angry" talk (DeCasper & Fifer, 1980; Menn & Stoel-Gammon, 1993) . The same researchers also documented the fact that newborns recognize many of the auditory stimuli that they have been previously exposed to *in utero*. For example, the youngest of babies have been shown to recognize their mothers' voices and to discriminate it from other voices that they hear. They have also been observed to recognize songs and the speech sounds that they were exposed to *in utero*.

Soon after birth, young babies also seem to be able to discriminate between utterances that are meant for them and those that are directed to other people. For example, a young baby might be playing intently with her mobile in her crib while, all around her, people are talking to one another. But if her mother turns toward the crib and says, "Hi, Susie, is everything OK? Are you having fun?" Susie will look toward her mother and "answer" with a smile and a cooing noise. The ability to recognize speech intended just for them continues to be observed among children throughout their early months and years. A 7-month-old Susie playing on the floor while adults seated around the room converse with each other will most often totally ignore the adult conversation. But if her mother says, "Honey, stop that—that's **not** what we do with our blocks," Susie will almost always stop her activity and look to her mother for clarification, more information, or instructions. A slight change in the inflectional pattern of her mother's speech, as well as her mother's change in the directionality of her utterance—away from the adults and toward her—alerted Susie to the fact that her mother's latest utterance was intended for her and not the other adults in the room.

The pervasive and distinctive way of talking to babies that occurs before birth naturally increases after birth when the mother finally gets the opportunity to interact face-to-face with her baby. In fact, the special style of talking to babies after birth involves not only mothers and other family members but many other nonfamily members as well. For example, psychologist Harriet Rheingold (Rheingold, 1973) reported a study in which she observed people in a hospital's nursery unit and discovered that nearly everyone (including the most senior physicians) stopped and talked to babies in the nursery in the same sing-songy, rhetorical manner that mothers use.

"And how are you today?" [pause] "Oh, what a nice smile. You feel good don't you? Are they treating you okay here in the nursery?"

"My, you're a sweet little girl. Where did you get all of that pretty hair?"

"Oh, you're awake. Did you have a nice nap? I'll bet you're hungry now, aren't you?"

The interesting thing is that most people who talk to newborns almost always pause as if they expect an answer from the baby. Thus, everyone, not just mothers, begins to demonstrate conversational patterns for children to hear beginning in the earliest days of infancy. Also, it is not just *adults* who offer these demonstrations. Young siblings of 4 and 5 years old will also hold these rhetorical "conversations" with newborns in the family. When talking with the new baby in their family, very young children will be heard using speech that reflects the same exaggerated intonations, pleasant melodic patterns, and pauses that characterize adults' speech to babies. Clearly, all of us who are around babies begin to involve them in the give-and-take pattern of human conversations months and months before they can begin to participate with their own speech.

## Making Newborn Babies "Communicators" Before They Understand the Nature of Communication

As social beings committed to interactions with other people, it is not natural for humans to be fully satisfied with these one-way conversations. Consequently, adults begin to act in ways that make these earliest one-way conversations feel as though they are two-way interactions. Research shows that mothers, fathers, other adults, and even older children who are around newborns make babies into communicators long before the baby understands the concept of communication (Bates, 1976; Sugarman-Bell, 1978). Adults accomplish this by carefully watching the baby's actions, eye-gaze, and emotional states and "assigning" communicative *meaning* to these actions and states. After assigning communicative meaning to a baby's actions, parents then respond to these meanings. By responding to their babies' actions as though they were intentional communicative acts, mature language users allow babies to have "communicative effects" on them months and months before the babies even begin to understand their power to communicate their *intentions* to others. You might hear a language specialist describe such a child as being in the *perlocutionary* stage of communicative development (Bates, 1976). Here are some common examples of this stage and the behavior on the part of parents and other adults around the child.

"I see your hand in your mouth. I'll bet you're hungry, aren't you?"

"Oh my, what a face! What's the matter? Are you uncomfortable? Are you wet? Let's see, no, it's not that. Tell me what's wrong. Oh, I see those sleepy eyes and that big yawn. You're sleepy, aren't you? Well, let's see if we can rock you to sleep."

"My what a nice smile. Are you happy? Do you like mamma to rub that lotion on you? Yes, that's what you like! Let's do it some more, okay?"

"I see you looking at that light. Say, 'I like that light.' Let's turn it off. Now let's turn it on. Isn't that a pretty light?"

"What are you looking at? Oh, your Teddy Bear. Do you want your Teddy? Mommy will get it for you. Here it is! Here's your nice Teddy. Yes, I can tell from your smile that that's what you wanted. Hug Teddy."

Such assignment of meaning and *communicative intentions* to a baby's nonlanguage behaviors reflects a downward extension of a society's rules for language use that we talked about in Chapter 1. Remember the rules?

1. Pay attention to another person's language utterance;

2. Try your best to understand what the speaker's intentions or desires are;

3. Do your best to respond to those intentions cooperatively and constructively.

Very young babies, of course, have no idea that their listeners are following these rules and are trying to respond to their "communicative intentions." In fact, as we have noted, very young babies do not yet understand the notion of having "intentions." In the first 4 or 5 months of life, babies' primary awareness is related to their general emotional and physical situations. For example, are they are comfortable or uncomfortable, happy or unhappy, hungry or sated? Is the object within their view (such as a lamp, mobile, or person) familiar or novel, interesting or uninteresting, or, perhaps, scary or friendly? Is an action being carried out (e.g., massaging him with lotion) pleasant or unpleasant? As a baby physically reacts to these varying states or emotions, caregivers interpret his or her actions and respond to them as though the baby had truly communicated some intention to them. In this way, caregivers make the most helpless of babies into communicators, almost from day one! For a review of the motor and cognitive development observed during babies' first 12 months, see Table 2–1. Babies respond to these inferred communicative intentions whenever it is possible for them to do so. After all, this is what people do for one another. We know this lesson well and we begin to practice it, instinctively and immediately, with our babies. Thus, even though the youngest babies are a long way from talking themselves, we talk to them with the language that we expect them to learn and use later in their development. In addition, as the examples above demonstrate, we make these interactions into *two-way conversations* by assigning meanings to babies' nonlanguage behaviors and states and then responding to the inferred meanings.

In the earliest stages of assignments of communicative intentions, babies can do little more than shift their gaze, smile, babble, and, though their body postures and facial expressions, reflect their relative state of comfort or discomfort. A bit later in their development, however, young babies gain the ability to use their motor movements to *act* on the entities of their environment. They become *proactive*. That is, they reach out and touch objects, grasp them, and throw them. They also reach out and touch people, push their hands away, and move away from events that are discomforting to them. The ability to physically act on the environment also comes before young babies understand the concept of *communication* and, certainly, long before they can produce language. Yet, the ability to physically act on

## Table 2-1
Development in Related Domains

| Age | Cognitive Developments | Motor Developments |
|-----|------------------------|--------------------|
| Birth | Visually prefers movement and contrasting visual patterns | Motor control begins developing from the head down |
| 1 month | Demonstrates regard for caregiver's face and nearby objects | Visual acuity is best within 8 inches from birth until 1 month |
| 2 months | Recognizes caregiver's face and anticipates objects' appearance | Achieves visual focus |
| 3 months | Visually searches for sources of actual sound | Reaches for and grasps objects |
| 4 months | Localizes sound sources; stares at place from which object was dropped | Establishes head control |
| 5 months | Recognizes familiar objects; explores objects through mouthing and touching | Sits up with slight support |
| 6 months | Enjoys dropping and picking up objects; shakes toys to make noises | Jaw control for chewing improves; grasps and transfers objects with both hands |
| 7 months | Imitates complex behaviors already achieved when able to view own performance | Crawls and pulls self to standing |
| 8 months | Prefers novel and relatively complex toys; unwraps wrapped objects | Manipulates objects and explores with index finger |
| 9 months | Uncovers hidden object if observes act of hiding; imitates familiar actions | Stands briefly with support and rolls into and out of sitting position |
| 10 months | Points to body parts on request; attains goal with trial-and-error approach | Makes stepping movements; holds and drinks from cup |
| 11 months | | Takes first independent steps |
| 12 months | Recognizes own name when called; imitates increasingly<br><br>Uses common objects appropriately; imitates movements not already in repertoire | Walks with one hand held; picks up objects with thumb-finger apposition |

Source: Adapted from Introduction to Language Development, by S. McLaughlin, 1998, pp. 177–178. San Diego, CA: Singular Publishing Group, Inc. Reprinted with permission.

entities provides caregivers with clearer signals of their baby's *intentions* and, thus, makes it easier for them to assign meanings to his or her actions.

The early conversational patterns and the assignment-of-meaning strategies used by adults with very young babies are more or less universal, although there are some interesting variations from culture to culture (Schieffelin & Eisenberg, 1984). In all cultures, however, parents and the other skilled language users who are around very young children have strong instincts for teaching both communication and language to babies. And, as we noted earlier, older children also quickly come to understand that this is a special teaching situation and they adopt the same kind of speech that they hear parents and other adults using with the new baby. Other children in a family will also begin to assign communicative intentions to their new sibling's behaviors. By watching the new babies' actions, the direction of their eye-gaze, and listening to their cries or cooing noises, older children will begin to respond to babies' perceived needs, just as parents and other adults do. Later, when these children grow up to be parents themselves, this style of talking to babies will be recalled and repeated as they begin to talk to their babies.

We need to be aware that all of this responsiveness by adults and older children is not unrewarded. The rewards, however, are social in nature and, thus, are not recognized and appreciated unless we think about them a bit. Playing out these responsive roles to develop their children's socialization and learning most often brings feelings of well-being and satisfaction in parents and other adults. These interactive roles of nurturing and teaching also bring caregivers much pure fun. Children's excitement, joy, and pleasure at being able to interact and satisfy their strong, innate drive to experience events and learn, bring equal joy and excitement to their caregivers. The fact that these activities are satisfying and fun for both babies and their caregivers is part of the grand plan that is inborn in most of us. This is why news reports about the abuse of babies are so disturbing to us. These cases reflect the actions of people who are behaving in ways that are absolutely contrary to normal instincts.

As we will discuss in later chapters, many aspects of modern life have effects on the opportunities and desires that people have to provide these important nurturative, teaching, and socializing interactions with children. We will discuss some research that indicates that, when babies' socialization activities are inadequate, children's later development in language and other important skill domains are negatively affected. As we will see when we elaborate on the overall early teaching and learning process, the final outcomes of a child's early social development and overall skill learning depend on *both* caregivers and babies playing their roles fully and skillfully.

## THE EARLY SOCIALIZATION OF VERY YOUNG CHILDREN

The earliest interactions of nurturing adults and very young infants that we have described to this point have focused on the efforts of the adults to be *responsive* to their infants' needs. However, for infants to develop further, they must be supported in becoming participants in their social environment. Thus, as babies develop physically, caregivers begin the process of helping infants develop the patterns of *interactions* that will prepare them for this participation.

### Establishing and Maintaining Interaction With Infants

In Chapter 1, we discussed the fact that people must interact with one another in cooperative ways in order to maintain societies that are secure and productive. Language, we saw, is the crucial element in fostering the complex, cooperative interactions needed to build advanced civilizations and cultures. It is logical, then, that language is taught and learned *in the context of human interactions*. Most parents instinctively understand that a key element in beginning to teach language is the creation and maintenance of nonlanguage, but social, interactions between their babies and themselves. Such interactions, are carried out by parents and others in the child's environment in parallel with their spoken "conversations" with them. This teaching of interaction, which also seems to be instinctive or recalled from previous experience, begins with adults seeking to establish two basic behavioral events with their babies: *joint attention* and *turn taking*. These two behaviors are taught to babies long before they learn language and they remain a part of their behavioral repertoires throughout their lives. In fact, you can recognize that, because they are a vital element in human interaction, they are also vital elements in our use of language. In our mature communicative patterns, we establish joint attention (a topic) and we take turns in our conversations.

## Joint Attention

Are you aware that every time we approach a very young infant, unless the baby is sleeping, we always look for ways to ensure that his or her attention is focused on us, on some object that we have in our possession, or something in the environment that we both can see and look at together? For example, most often, we approach a baby so that we are in line with the baby's line of vision. We put ourselves directly in front of the infant. If we want the baby's attention on us, we put our faces close to his or hers. We talk to our babies as we approach them. If their attention is focused elsewhere, we make little noises or touch them so that their focus shifts to us. We smile and caress them. Often, we bring them a small object and move it into their line of vision. Usually, we try to bring an object that is active or interesting in some way. Perhaps it's shiny or soft or makes a noise. We might hold babies' nursing bottles in front of their eyes and touch their lips with them—talking to them all the while

If babies do not respond to our efforts to interact with them, it is usually a sign that they are distracted or fatigued. Sometimes, however, adult efforts to evoke interactive responses from babies are a bit overzealous and our attempts to interact are overstimulating to them. Research indicates that adult caregivers are generally sensitive to a baby's signals (Snow & Ferguson, 1979). If we judge that the baby's nonresponsiveness is because of his or her distraction, we look to see what's competing with us. Is the infant looking at something else? If so, we adopt the infant's "line-of-regard" and also look at the object or activity he or she is focused on. We begin to talk about the object of the child's gaze. Touch it if it is near. We might even bring the object of his or her regard closer so that he or she can reach out and touch it. If the object of our joint attention with the baby is a noisemaker, we squeeze it, shake it, or rewind it so that the noise continues. Then we make whatever effort it takes to maintain this process of jointly attending to something for at least some short period of time.

When we judge that a baby's resistance to our efforts at interaction are a result of his or her fatigue or because our efforts are overstimulating, we are sensitive to these signals and generally will stop or tone down the interaction. If, however, we judge the infant's resistance to be simply a loss of interest in the object at hand, we will search for a new focus for joint attention and maintain this new interaction as long as the child wishes to. This establishing of "joint focus" with the very young infant seems to be a universal instinct—everyone does it. Why? The reason is simple and yet critical: *We cannot interact with another person unless each of us is focused on one another, or unless both of us share a joint focus on some other nearby object, action, or event.* Quite simply, we must have something, a *topic* to interact around.

Think about it. Why are cocktail party conversations with strangers so difficult? Most often it is because we have no joint focus or topic to converse about with people with whom we have no history of interaction. What do we do in these situations? If we desire to make conversation at all, we try to establish some topic or joint focus of attention so that we can interact around it. Thus, we might comment on the food we are sharing. "Have you tried the ham roll-ups? They're delicious." It is common in Western cultures to try to establish some shared topic around one another's personal circumstances; thus we might ask, "Are you a business associate of the hosts? No, well what business are you in? Oh, you're a teacher. What do you teach? English? Well, I'd better watch my grammar. I'm an attorney myself." "What grade do you teach? My son is a seventh grader and is having a tough time in English." Having found a topic of common interest and experience, these two strangers can now construct a meaningful conversation.

As we establish various topics, items, or information around which we can begin to weave conversations or interactions with others, we begin to feel more comfortable and integrated into the party. "Here, let me hold your drink while you put a plate of these goodies together. Do you practice civil or criminal law? I've always been intrigued with criminal law." And so we are able to function appropriately through an often long, long night by understanding the rules and requirements of human interactions.

Because we understand that a joint focus on some object, action, state, or event is critical to human interactions, we establish this fact early with our youngest infants. We help them learn it by doing it. As adults skilled in interactions, we use all of our knowledge to maintain our babies in periods of interaction with us. We play "Chase" ("I'm going to get you!"). We make rattles rattle. We make music boxes play. We make toy cars "go." We make balls roll to the child. We trade hugs and kisses. We carry them around a room to look at things—"See the kitty? Nice kitty. Pet the kitty. No, not too rough now—like this (strokes kitten) pet, pet, pet. That's better!" All of these activities serve to establish some joint focus around which we can both interact in some positive, constructive way. Early on, with very young babies, adults do most of the work in these interactions. Children's early contributions to these interactions most often consist of *reactions* to the adult's activities. They squeal, laugh, and wave their arms as we carry out these little rituals with them. Gradually, though, babies seek to play a more *proactive* role in the games. They reach and take the rattle; they shake it, mouth it, and then give it back to the adult. They attempt to roll the ball. They turn the pages of a book the adult is sharing with them. Throughout the developmental stages of early infancy, adults use these interactive occasions to demonstrate to very young children the kinds of activities that are suited to different types of objects. It is in these contexts that children learn to roll and throw balls, shake rattles, pet animals carefully, turn cranks on jack-in-the-boxes, and push the switch so that action toys and music boxes can perform their functions.

### Cooperative Turn Taking

As we take our small interactions around a common focus, we begin to extend them into longer and, hopefully, more meaningful routines. We do so by creating a turn-taking pattern. Turn taking is the glue that connects individual bits of human interaction and combines them into whole episodes of interactions that, at some point, end in a result that is fun or productive for the parties involved. Games are played. Turns are traded in peek-a-boo, putting blocks in a can, or rolling a ball to one another. We take turns stacking blocks into towers. Later, houses and garages are built by taking turns placing blocks.

Cooperative turn taking is the pattern we follow in all of our communicative, work, and play interactions. If turn taking is not forthcoming in an interaction with someone, we become annoyed and feel left out. After all, if the root of human interactions is *cooperative* in nature, not allowing a partner a turn to make his or her contribution to the interaction violates the rules of the interaction process to which we are all committed. So it is that we begin to show our interacting infants the "rules of the turn-taking game," and we begin to do so quite early in infancy.

Remember, adults talking to newly born babies usually pause after each comment or question to leave room for the baby to respond, even though they know that the baby cannot talk. Remember also, adults' instincts to take any response that the baby makes and treat it as though the baby had responded meaningfully to their utterance. For example, we say, "How are you today?" Then we pause and take a child's "coo," smile, squeal, or fussing behavior as our answer and proceed to take another turn for ourselves. "That's good. I think your nap helped, didn't it? (pause) Are you ready for a bottle? (pause) Okay, mamma's got one all ready for you. Here it is! Oh, you were ready for that weren't you? Yes, yes indeed."

Later, as children become more skilled in their ability to attend to and manipulate objects, we apply the same strategy. We do something to the object and wait. For example, we might put a block in a can and wait. Children are great imitators, so the probability is high that, if they can pick up and release a small block, they will follow suit and drop a block in the can also. We then praise the child, "Good girl," and we will then repeat our action and wait again for the baby to take his or her turn. If children cannot imitate the action we demonstrate, we will often take their hands and physically "put them through" the act. On the other hand, if a child continues to put blocks in the can, ignoring the adult partner, we may interrupt, draw the child's attention, and say something like, "Wait—let Mommy take her turn now." (Mother takes turn.) "Now, it's your turn." Here we see that teaching turn-taking means that we are teaching *two* acts:

1. Fill your turn

2. Wait your next turn by allowing a turn from your partner

Thus, we set up interactions that allow the child to learn and follow the rules of human interaction. Again, we have structured a situation that allows the child to discover a skill by practicing it with someone who already knows and uses it. Therefore, like most of the teaching we have been describing as occurring at this early level, the instruction in turn taking uses the technique of allowing children to *learn by doing.*

When we have helped children to learn to adopt and maintain a common focus and fill and wait turns with a partner, we have established the rudimentary pattern of *joint* human interactions through which everything else can be learned. We have established the first and most basic social skill. We then take this basic interaction skill and apply it in every situation that we possibly can. We immerse our children in interactive jointly focused, turn-taking routines that end in all sorts of results, We set up routines such as "Chase," "peek-a-boo," and "you-take-one-and-I'll-take-one" that *regulate one another's actions.* We look through books and take turns pointing at the animals that the adult names and, thus, we *regulate one another's attention.* We take turns winding the jack-in-the-box until the clown suddenly pops out of the box. We give and take objects from one another with both saying *thank you* after each exchange. As the child develops further, we pour and drink our drinks at a pretend tea party. We "cook dinner" by pretending to pour, stir, and ladle. We play out simple caregiving routines with dolls. Table 2–2 summarizes the types of interactive routines that emerge during early childhood. As you can see, the routines become more complex and more social as children demonstrate that they are ready for more complexity. As we will see later in this chapter, these routines also provide the ideal context for babies to learn to comprehend and produce language.

As you can see from the variety of these early interactions, it is within these repeating routines that we begin to *teach* our children the important skills that they will need to interact successfully in both their *physical* and their *social* worlds. Once again, our babies are "learning by doing" because we, as skilled, socialized adults, are setting up interactive scenarios that allow us to demonstrate and reward the kinds of behaviors that we know our children will need. Our infants soak up these experiences and slowly but surely build behavioral repertoires that will allow them to interact successfully with any of the other people in their environments, as well as perform appropriately on the many aspects of their physical world.

### Table 2-2

Adult-Directed Contexts for Teaching the Socialization Skills That Will Faciltate All Early Learning

---

- *Establish* **basic interaction episodes:**

  Establish and maintain *joint attention* with child
  Establish and maintain *joint actions* with child
  Establish *turn-taking* and *turn waiting*

- *Extend* **interactive episodes into oft-repeated** *routines*

  With very young babies play extended rounds of games such as:

  Peek-a-boo
  Chase
  Where is it?—Here it is!

  With babies of 6 to 10 months, develop interactive *turn-taking* routines such as:

  Building with blocks
  Simple doll-play (feed, rock-the-baby, etc.)
  Book-reading where child points to pictures named
  Car and truck scenarios (run, back-up, park)
  Large child puzzles and toy mailboxes for various shaped blocks

  With toddlers of 10 to 24 months play out *product producing* scenarios such as:

  Building things with blocks or Legos
  Preparing snacks (S'Mores, toast and jelly, etc,)
  Assembling break-apart cars, trucks, helicopters
  Drawing and coloring

  Also with toddlers and older children, play out *social scenarios* such as:

  Tea party, house, school, store, doctor, etc.
  Pretend cooking
  Extended doll play (bathe, dress, feed, etc.)

  With preschoolers of 3 to 5 years begin to play rule-bound games

  Card games
  Board games
  Read books
  Play video games

---

The very basic social skills being discovered in these interactive scenarios are those that we identified in Chapter 1, which Bruner (1975) classified as "people skills." Learning such skills goes on for a lifetime as we learn more and more sophisticated ways to interact successfully with other people. As you can anticipate, such skills will eventually encompass everything from proper language, appropriate politeness and etiquette to skills in humor, persuasion, and overall constructiveness. In many ways, our people skills form the core of what others might call our "personality," and later, our relative popularity, our leadership potential, and our overall sociability.

Clearly, these interactive activities also provide babies with opportunities to perform skilled actions on the real things in their environment—building blocks, wind-up toys, tools, cooking and eating utensils, books, pull-toys, TVs, tape players, and hundreds of other objects. Thus, in parallel to gaining people skills, babies are also learning important behavioral repertoires for operating on this physical world—a general repertoire that Bruner (1975) has called "thing skills." The latter skills, along with people skills, also become lifelong learning tasks as our children grow and learn the many specialized actions needed to make all of the entities in their world perform appropriately and productively. We will discuss the specific "thing skills" that children discover in more detail in Chapter 5. Meanwhile, we offer Table 2–3, which summarizes some of the key adult interactive strategies for helping a child to discover the early "thing skills" that start them on the road to gaining the rich, physical-world knowledge they will need.

## Using Joint Action Routines to Enhance an Infant's Socialization Skills

Another part of preparing our infants to live in their social world of other people lies in helping them to discover, value, and trust that the other people in their environment will follow the rules of interaction by responding to them promptly and co-operatively. Obviously, newborn babies develop strong attachments to their mothers and other primary caregivers who feed them, soothe them, and cuddle them. This emotional attachment is the base for a child's eventual understanding of the notion of a social world in which other people are separate from themselves and are the sources for sensual (cuddling, caressing, rocking, rubbing, feeding) and sensory (speech, noise, smells, objects to touch) stimulation.

Child development research consistently supports the importance of an infant's early interactions, and the establishment

## Table 2-3

Adult Strategies for *Facilitating* the Development of Young Children's Knowledge of the Physical World

---

- Respond positively to children's actions on toys and objects
- Demonstrate how to play with a variety of toys
- Demonstrate what to do with various objects in environment
- Allow child time and provide materials for solo exploration and experimentation with "things" (toy tools, action toys, pots and pans, paper and crayons, toy sets with animals, toy cars and trucks, "busy boxes," etc.)
- "Scaffold" (Bruner, 1975) for the child. Do the first parts of a complex (or long chain) of actions and let the child perform the *last* action. Here are three examples:

    Turn the crank on the jack-in-the-box until it is ready to "pop-up," and then let the child make the action-producing last turn of the crank;

    Stack-up lower blocks, and let child put on the "topper" on the tower;

    Wind-up the music box and let the child push the switch that turns it on;

    Place the first pieces of the large puzzle and let the child set the last piece that completes it;

    After several episodes of such "scaffolding" start doing less of the action and let the child do a little more each time until he or she can complete the entire action chain.
- Let the child "show-off" his or her skills with toys and household objects—wait, and restrain yourself from "helping" until the child shows a real need for help.
- Show obvious approval of child's skills and inventiveness.
- Have fun and make sure it is fun for the child—this is not life or death and the child does not have to do everything perfectly.
- "Stretch" the child by introducing more and more complex materials and scenarios into the routines.
- Talk about what you are doing. Match your words to the object or action that is immediately salient to the child.

---

of secure attachments for later cognitive and emotional development (Honig, 1993). In fact, studies of early neurological development suggest that positive interactions between infants and their caregivers stimulate the release of chemicals in the child's brain that support the formation of increasingly elaborate neural networks. When circumstances interfere with the attainment of true attachment between babies and their caregivers, problems, ranging from emotional instability to learning problems, can occur throughout life.

When successful experiences and interactions with caregivers occur, infants learn that other people are ready and willing to respond to them. As they find both success and pleasure in their participation in the interactive routines offered by their caregivers, babies cross the threshold of socialization. While infants remain highly self-centered in their search for comfort and well-being, they also begin to indicate their strong drive to be with and interact with the other important people in their environment. They have begun to learn, as their ancient forebearers did, that their well-being is dependent on the cooperation of others. Thus, other people become the demonstrators and models for the behaviors they must acquire. From this point on into adulthood, then, children seek to acquire both the social and the sensorimotor skills that their adult models demonstrate for them.

The interactions in which adults engage young babies are noteworthy because they model the give and take, turn-taking patterns that characterize all human interaction, including language exchanges. These early, often-repeated interactions were termed "joint action routines" by Bruner (1975). Through their responding and waiting in these interactions, caregivers show children that they are expected to participate in social exchanges. In the earliest interactive routines, such as "peek-a-boo" and other such early rituals, the adult carries the bulk of the activity and produces all of the language. All that is expected is that the child will react—hopefully, happily, with a big smile and a laugh. Babies love these little reciprocal routines and will often keep an adult "peeking" and "chasing" them for periods far longer than most adults really want to play. But, most of the time, adults will continue to play as long as the child will respond.

Importantly, however, if children tire of the game and begin to look away and quit responding, the adult will usually stop the game immediately. Caregivers understand that these early social exchanges must be kept happy and interesting or it defeats their purpose of getting children to look on other people as sources of pleasure, comfort, and responsiveness. Babies let us know when we are overdoing our interactions with them by denying us their attention. They look away from us and sometimes cry or fuss. Usually, adults are sensitive to these actions and assign communicative significance to them, saying such things as:

"Oh, you're tired of that game, huh? Well, would you like me to walk you around a bit or would you like to play with your music box?"

"I see that you're more interested more in what your brother's doing than me. Okay, we'll play my game later."

"Oh my, you're so fussy. Let's have a bottle and a nap and then we'll play our game."

As these joint action routines continue and children become more and more mature and skilled at participating in them, adults begin to use them to show the child all of the rewards that human interactions can provide for them. Routines begin to be focused on interactions that produce some highly desirable end results. For example, cooking and eating routines teach children to learn to pour drinks, stir with spoons, and "serve" imaginary hamburgers and cake. The same routines set the context for children to acquire proper manners for requesting items from others and acknowledging the other person's helpful response. Such routines also allow them the opportunities needed to learn turn-taking communicative interaction patterns that will finally attain a level that we call "conversation." Routines that are structured around toy barns, fences, and farm animals provide children opportunities to learn that animals eat, drink, make distinctive noises, and sleep. They also learn that some animals are called "cows" and others are called by different names such as "horses," "pigs," or "doggies." In other interactive scenarios, books are used to structure stories about people and their life activities. In still other play contexts, rudimentary physics is taught by working together to put things together or making certain items "work." It is in these actions on the environment that children learn that, if one wants to put a block in a cup, the block must be smaller than the cup, or that if a music box or toy car is to run, it must be "wound-up." In such interactive play, children have more experiences that reinforce their awareness that the adults around them are good bets for helping them carry out a difficult task that they haven't yet mastered and for providing other supportive acts, such as seeing that the toys that need to be wound up are, indeed, wound up. This knowledge about the supportive and constructive role that adults are committed to playing with them is a key factor in children's eventual discovery that they can have certain effects on adult behaviors through certain of their own actions. This discovery, of course, is the key element in children's later discovery and implementation of *intentions* to have effects on the others around them through issuance of communicative acts. The emergence and refinement of nonverbal but intentional communicative acts will be covered in more detail in Chapter 5.

## Joint Action Routines as a Context for Language Learning

Besides being the context for all sorts of nonverbal learning by babies, it is in the "joint action routines" that caregivers also begin to put their language behaviors into the specific (and highly salient) contexts that will help their children to comprehend the meanings of various words and phrases used by the people around them. It is in such routines that children begin to learn the "names" of the hundreds of entities and actions in their environment. Also, it is in these routines that they hear the names of events such as bye-bye, beddy-time, mommy's home, and "states," such as hungry, sleepy, all gone, and more . It is in these routines that language is broken down into child-sized bits and used to refer to things and events that the child is experiencing at the time the words or phrases are used. Because these routines are repeated time after time and become quite familiar to the child, they offer intensive teaching occasions.

### Adult Talk Is About the Here and Now

What joint action routines allow, from the very beginning and throughout the early childhood years, is talk to young children that is focused on things and actions that are immediate to the context of their interactions. Because young babies have no concept of past and future times, we must initially concentrate on teaching language elements that refer to the objects and actions that the baby is seeing and feeling while he or she is hearing the words and phrases. This is referred to as talking about things that are "here and now." Thus, we give the baby the opportunity of hearing the "names" of things and actions used at the same time as he or she is experiencing them. Because we carry out these favorite interactive routines many, many times with our babies, we soon find that they are able to hear a word and understand, at least grossly, what it refers to. Thus, when we say "peek-a-boo" 6-month-old babies will put their hands over their eyes or pull their blankets over their heads. Babies are developing an ability to comprehend many of the words they are hearing. They are developing what is called a "receptive vocabulary." They are beginning to understand words spoken to them several months before they will actually produce their first word.

## INCREASING THE USE OF WORDS TO HAVE EFFECTS ON BABIES' BEHAVIOR

As caregivers see that babies are beginning to comprehend some of the words spoken to them, they begin to shift into serious language teaching. They branch out a bit in both the specific words they use and in the meanings these words have. By this we mean that parents, realizing that their words can now have effects on children's behavior, begin to broaden the role of words in a child's environment. There seem to be three broad areas in which parents in Western cultures almost always begin to work with their children. The first is the use of words to assure the *safety* of their children. Thus, words like "No-No!" "Hot!" "Stop!" "Ugh, dirty, dirty!" are used very early. These obviously are most needed at the beginning of the stage when children begin to crawl and then walk—typically, around 7 to 12 months. The second area of early word teaching involves the development of a vocabulary of "referential" or "substantive" words. These are the crucial words that *refer to* or *name* objects, actions, and states in the environment. Somewhat surprisingly, another area in which parents concentrate their word teaching is in the area of *politeness* terms. They begin to use words such as "Thank you, "Excuse me," and "Please" with their children. Remember, at these early stages of language teaching, these words are being taught in a "receptive" mode. That is, parents use them at every opportunity, hoping to help the child learn to "comprehend" them. Adults do not expect the child to produce these words at this point. Thus, when a baby hands mother his favorite toy, a mother might say, "Thank you— I love your Teddy bear. He's so soft." Caregivers routinely use "Please" with requests to their children. "Please give me a kiss."

"Please stop that." "Will you please come here." "May I please have your spoon?" The fourth area of early word-teaching is in an area referred to by Nelson (1973) as "expressive words." These are words such as "Whoops," "Oh, Oh," and "Wheee" that usually mark events or actions that are fun or happy.

As care providers use words, they are teaching at several different levels. First, they are trying to help children learn what certain words *refer to*. They do this by emphasizing the use of words that refer to entities, actions, and events that are in the immediate context of their interactions with the children. Secondly, care providers are intent on beginning to demonstrate what words are supposed to *do* in the world, that is, to *have effects* on those to whom they are addressed. Thus, in addition to teaching words that allow caregivers and children to *refer* to things, they also begin to teach a number of words that directly regulate another person's behaviors, such as the "safety" words we mentioned and the politeness words and phrases that we have identified. Parents invest considerable time and effort in teaching children to comprehend and respond appropriately to these important words and short phrases.

Safety words, such as *No, No, stop*, and *don't* are usually spoken loudly and abruptly and children usually react to them by immediately stopping whatever they are doing and looking at the mother or father who spoke to them. Of course, this is exactly the effect that we want these words to have. Politeness words and expressive words, in contrast, are most often said sweetly and with exaggerated inflections. As a result, children's reactions are usually pleasant ones. They laugh and, more often than not, repeat whatever they were doing that evoked these words. Have you ever had the experience of smiling and saying "Thank you" in an exaggerated way when a child gave you something—and then been caught up in an interaction in which you were uttering a string of "Thank yous" as the child gave you everything he or she could lay hands on?

Some of the words adults use in these contexts are more "abstract" than others. That is, their referent is not as tangible as the "name" of a toy or action. These include politeness words as well as many of our language's "little" words such as *in, of, this, that, my*, and *why*. Thus, adults begin using many of these very early with children. We know, for example, that it will take a lot of experience with the words before children can fully understand exactly what "please," "excuse me," and "thank you" mean. Other such abstract words are probably only truly learned by using them. In fact, when children begin to say these words themselves at around 1 year of age, they use them in exactly the same situations in which their language-teaching caregivers used them—probably still not fully understanding them but figuring that they were important or mother would not have said them so often. Gradually, by observing their partners' responses to these words, they begin to form ideas about the words' meanings. A young child's use of words such as "Thank-oo," "Oh Oh," or "why" also usually evokes very positive reactions from the adults around them. It is at this point that children begin to understand that words have real power in their world. If mere, but specific "mouth noises" like these can evoke a smile and a hug from one of those big people around them, children are only too happy to oblige and produce them. In a very real and powerful way, caregivers have taught their child that words are *acts on other people and that other people will respond to them.* If this is true, a child might reason, there is every reason for them to begin to consistently listen, respond to, and learn the words and phrases that are directed to them.

## CHILDREN BECOME INTENTIONAL COMMUNICATORS: THEY LEARN THAT THEY CAN HAVE EFFECTS ON OTHER PEOPLE'S BEHAVIORS

### The Emergence of Communicative Intentions

We will look at what the child learns through each of these various early stages of development in more detail in Chapter 5. However, it is necessary here to anticipate some aspects of this learning in order to discuss a few of the specific changes in children's behavior. These changes are important in alerting parents to develop additional sensitivities and strategies in their interactions with babies. It is the caregivers' responsibility to stay closely tuned in to their children's learning because they must make important adjustments in the style and content of their interactive activities and language usage to help children move onto the next major learning level.

Thus, at about the same time that children begin to understand and respond to words and phrases directed to them, they also begin to show us that they finally understand the most basic rudiments of social "communication." Shortly before they begin to produce words, babies indicate that they have discovered that they can, through their nonlanguage actions, have effects on other people. Remember that, up to this point, parents and others around the child have been interpreting the child's behaviors and *assigning* meaning to them. Thus, adults have been making the child into a communicator by being sensitive and responding to his or her nonverbal states and actions. At around 9 to 12 months of age, however, typically developing children reach a crucial stage in which they begin to produce nonlanguage behaviors that are specifically communicative, that is, behaviors *directed toward* people around them and *intended* to evoke some response from these people. In Chapter 5 we will consider the details of this breakthrough in child skills. For now, however, we will simply discuss this breakthrough in general fashion.

We need to emphasize the point that children's demonstration of *intentions to communicate does not mean that they begin to use language.* It simply means that they have discovered that they can have effects on *people* through their own actions. This discovery emerges soon after children discover the sensorimotor concept of *mean-to-desired-ends* with physical objects. The discovery of the *means-ends* concept means that children have discovered that they can anticipate a result from their own action. They can open and empty a can of building blocks and stack them. They can then slap at the tower and knock all of the blocks down. They can tug on the string of their toy duck and make it move along behind them while it produces the *quacking* sounds typical of that toy. When the *means-to-ends* concept is applied to people, it means that children now know, for example, that if they look at and touch or reach toward an object—their interactive adult partner will likely follow their lead and manipulate and talk about that object. When they realize this "power" to have *effects* on the behaviors of others, babies will perform an act on an object and then *wait* for a partner's response to their action.

As you can deduce from these examples, children first communicate without language through the use of motor acts on people and things. Babies tug on adults and throw an unwanted toy. They use *body language*, such as pulling away or moving to closer proximity to their partner. They posture in ways that signal their happy anticipation of some expected action of their adult partner. We have all observed a child sitting upright with eyes on us and more-or-less rocking with excitement as we prepared to complete a routine that is well-known by the child.

## The Emergence of Communicative Gestures

At this point, children begin to use rudimentary communicative *gestures,* such as open-hand requests; reaching movements that indicate a request for an object that is some distance away or a request that the adult attend to that distant object; holding out an object to "show" it to an adult; holding out an object for the adult to take and act on in some way; and bye-bye waves. The final gesture learned is the one-finger pointing gesture that is used in many different ways. The development of gestures is a fascinating process that we will examine carefully and in detail, This development is one of the child's learning domains that we will detail in Chapter 5. Suffice to say here, when intentions to act so as to have effects on people emerge, it is a major milestone and a truly momentous event. Our babies have become *communicators*—able to act on us directly and purposefully to attain objects, states, and activities that they desire. They are embarking on a journey that will take them through several stages in the development of the specific and specialized behaviors that are designed for human communication. This development, of course, will typically culminate in a fully developed speech and language system. Their world, and ours, has changed forever.

In Chapter 3, we continue to discuss the actions and strategies parents and other caregiving adults use as they adjust their focus to include support and teaching of their children's production of spoken language.

## SUMMARY

- Parents and others in developing infants' environment play a key role in their early socialization.

- Mothers' talk to their unborn babies and new infants is so unique it has been given a special name: motherese or parentese.

- Parents, adults, and siblings begin to involve babies in the give-and-take pattern of human communication long before they can talk. They talk to babies as if they will respond and assign meaning to babies' nonlanguage behaviors and states.

- Parents create and maintain nonlanguage, social interactions with their babies and through them teach two important social behaviors: joint attention and turn taking. These behaviors are repeated naturally in parents' interaction with babies in joint action routines.

- The talk that goes on during joint action routines is simplified for the child and focuses on the here and now, rather than the past or future.

- As babies develop, parents use more words to describe and control their babies' behavior. As parents use more words to affect behavior, babies and toddlers learn that words can have effects on other people.

- Before babies can use language, they reach a crucial stage of development in which they produce behaviors (acting on things and people) that are intended to get a response from people in their environment. This basic, nonlanguage communication develops further into communicative gestures.

## References

Bates, E. (1976). *Language and context*. New York: Academic Press.

Bruner, J. S. (1975). The ontogenesis of speech acts. *Journal of Child Language, 2*, 1–19.

DeCasper, A. J., & Fifer, W. P. (1980). Of human bonding: Newborns prefer their mothers' voices. *Science, 208*, 1174–1176.

Honig, A. S. (1993). Mental health for babies: What do theory and research teach us? *Young Children, 48*(3), 69–76.

Menn, L., & Stoel-Gammon, C. (1993). Phonological development: Learning sounds and sound patterns. In J. B. Gleason (Ed.), *The development of language* (pp. 65–114). New York: Macmillan.

Nelson, K. (1973). Structure and strategy in learning to talk. *Monographs of the Society for Research in Child Development, 38*(No. 149).

Rheingold, H. (1973). The effect of environmental stimulation upon social and exploratory behavior. In L. J. Stone, H. T. Smith, & L. B. Murphy (Eds.), *The competent infant* (pp. 789–795). New York: Basic Books.

Schieffelin, B. B., & Eisenberg, A. R. (1984). Cultural variation in children's conversations. In R. Schiefelbusch & J. Pickar (Eds.), *The acquisition of communicative competence* (Vol. 8, pp. 377–420). Baltimore: University Park Press.

Snow, C. E., & Ferguson, C. A. (Eds.). (1979). *Talk to children: Language input and acquisition.* Cambridge, UK: Cambridge University Press.

Sugarman-Bell, S. (1978). Some organizational aspects of pre-verbal communication. In J. Markova (Ed.), *The social context of language* (pp. 49–66). New York: John Wiley.

# THE ROLE OF PARENTS AND OTHER ADULTS IN TEACHING LANGUAGE TO YOUNG CHILDREN

## JAMES McLEAN

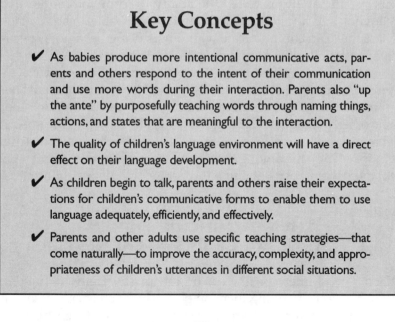

## Key Concepts

✔ As babies produce more intentional communicative acts, parents and others respond to the intent of their communication and use more words during their interaction. Parents also "up the ante" by purposefully teaching words through naming things, actions, and states that are meaningful to the interaction.

✔ The quality of children's language environment will have a direct effect on their language development.

✔ As children begin to talk, parents and others raise their expectations for children's communicative forms to enable them to use language adequately, efficiently, and effectively.

✔ Parents and other adults use specific teaching strategies—that come naturally—to improve the accuracy, complexity, and appropriateness of children's utterances in different social situations.

## INTRODUCTION

In the preceding chapter we discussed the role of adults in socializing their very young infants. We saw that adults bring children into their social world by structuring the patterns of human interaction that are basic to a social world. Thus, babies learn to interact cooperatively and productively with the other people in their environment by following the "rules" basic to human interactions.

We have also seen how parents and other care-giving adults talk to their children. In this talk, they model the linguistic elements of the language of their particular segment of our overall culture. They carefully structure interactions and modulate their talking in ways that bring the words and phrases they use into juxtaposition with the entities, people, relationships, states, and actions that are in the immediate context in which they are interacting with their children. In these contexts, babies learn to *comprehend* many of the words and phrases of the spoken language of their culture and match them up with their *referents.*

In the final stages of this process we also saw that young babies attain a level of social skills in which they fully understand the fact that they can affect the behaviors of other people. In other words, they can intentionally act on others to satisfy some need. This specific ability is called the ability to form communicative intentions and apply them to others. In fact, babies reach a stage where they can communicate with others using behaviors specifically designed for communication—gestures.

At this point, as happens throughout children's early development, parents and other adults in children's environments begin to alter their behaviors toward children. In addition to all of their other interactions and teaching, adults now include special behaviors and strategies to support the development of true, symbolic language among their child learners. In this chapter, we will discuss this transition in adult behaviors toward children.

## THE TEACHING OF SPOKEN
## LANGUAGE BEGINS IN EARNEST

When a child intentionally acts on others physically by tugging at their hand or handing them an object, he or she has crossed an important milestone. When he or she begins to make gestures directed toward another and expects a response to these gestures, the child has moved to yet a different level of communicative skill. Realizing that the child has moved up to a higher and more effective communicative level, adults around the child also shift their own behaviors upward to another level.

Parents understand that *the next step up* from these intentionally communicative motor acts that adults are expected to *respond to* will be acquiring a system of true symbolic language. Adults recognize when language is the next step to be anticipated from a child, because they are intuitively alert to several child behavioral indicators. First, children begin to issue more and more specific communicative acts. They also begin to use fewer physical actions on their partners and produce more and more gestures directed toward their partners. Importantly, children also begin to produce more and more vocalizations with their gestures. They signal urgency or impatience with their vocalizations. After only few weeks at the gestural level, parents realize that their child's communicative desires and needs are far *beyond* those that he or she can adequately express through gestures, even when the gestures are supplemented by nonlanguage vocalizations. Parents begin to see frustration in the child's efforts to express his or her desires and they begin to be frustrated themselves. "Just what is it that you want?" a mother might say after making two or three honest efforts to understand a child's communicative gestural acts. At this point both mothers and children understand that it is time to move on to a more effective and efficient way of communicating and both begin to move toward that better system—*spoken language*. The shift in caregiver behavior, as others before it, usually begins just before the child has arrived at the absolute point of readiness to learn spoken language and, in a way, "primes" the child's readiness levels. As we will see in Chapter 4, children work mightily to learn—and to learn *how* to learn.

In anticipation of the next developmental stage of learning spoken language, then, parents and others around babies do two specific things:

1. They respond readily and positively to their children's intentional communicative acts, which are now at the nonverbal level of motor acts on things and people and gestures;

**2.** They begin to feed children an increasing diet of new words to help prepare them for the next level in which they will begin to produce words themselves.

At this point, too, caregivers fully expect that their children will respond to their words and they begin to insist that they do by repeating their message or, if they perceive that the child did not understand it, by modifying it in some way. The latter strategy is called "repairing" a message, and speakers do this throughout their lives when they feel that a message has been misunderstood. In the course of repairing a message, parents and other caregivers keep their words simple and their sentences, while complete, are not too long or too complex. They want their children to hear the words clearly and they want these words and/or phrases to stand out from all of the other language that surrounds the child.

It is at this point (typically between 10 and 12 months of age) that children begin to be specifically "instructed" about how to produce language. This is the point where things, actions, and states (e.g., happy, sad, hungry) are always named. In most homes, picture books come out and adults give animals, people, and objects "names." After a few weeks of this "feeding" of language to children, they also begin to encourage children to try to produce the words themselves.

"Here is the cow. Point to the cow. What does the cow say? It says Mooo. Say, 'Mooo.'"

"Where is the Mama bear? Where is the baby bear? What are they doing? Yes, they are eating. They are eating their dinner. Who is this? Right, it's baby bear!"

"Where is your Teddy bear? Go get mama your Teddy bear. No, that's your bunny. Go get your Teddy bear. Yes, that's your Teddy bear. Nice Teddy bear. Say 'nice Teddy.'"

"Do you want a bite of mama's cookie? Yes. Just take one bite (holds up one finger). That's it. Take one bite. Oh, isn't that good? Yummy, Yummy. Do you want more? Say, 'more please.'"

"Uh oh, you spilled your milk. Let's wipe that up okay? Wipe, wipe. There, it's all clean. But your milk is all gone. Milk is all gone (shows empty glass). Let's get some more milk. Say 'More milk.' There, now you have more milk. Say 'thank you.'"

Notice that the adult talk is still about "here and now" objects and actions. *The Three Bears* picture book is open and each thing named is pointed to. The Teddy bear is real and at hand. The one bite of cookie is, indeed, *yummy*. The milk is *spilled*; it is, indeed, *all gone*; and *more* milk is made available.

As such talk goes on and adult-requested words are produced more often by the child, caregivers begin to pause to leave more room for a child to act and talk. At first, the child's actions are simply to point to the picture, the Teddy bear or the milk. Soon, however, children also begin to use the words that are being fed to them. They will repeat the key words that the caregiver has emphasized by exaggerated voice inflections and frequent repetitions. At this stage, the child's pronunciation will probably not be too accurate; but rough approximations are readily accepted by their partners. In Chapter 6, when we look at the child's specific language learning products during this developmental period, we will look in more detail at the emergence of early speech sounds and early vocabularies of typically developing children. In this chapter devoted to looking at caregiver behaviors and their teaching, however, it is interesting to note that a caregiver's speaking "style" shows up immediately in children's earliest spoken words. For example, the previously cited research by psycholinguist Katherine Nelson (1973) shows that some caregivers are more "expressive" than others. Their speech includes many words that refer to emotions rather than to specific objects or actions. Such a parent might use a lot of utterances such as "Whoops we go!" "Wheee!" "Oh Oh!" "I love you, you darling!" "Oh, please, please, please!" "Wow!"

Other parents are more what Nelson calls "referential." These parents tend to concentrate on so-called substance words that *refer* to or *name* specific things and actions: "This is a birdy— say birdy." "What's the boy doing? He's running—run, run, run little boy." Of course, all parents do some of *both* kinds of word teaching. As we should expect, however, the vocabularies of children of highly enthusiastic or emotional parents have been shown to use more "expressive" words; while children of more matter-of-fact caregivers tend to have finely tuned "referential" word vocabularies for talking about objects and actions in the world and usually use fewer emotional words. From these data, we can see clearly that what children learn about language at home is what they will use early in their own spoken language.

An extensive research study by Hart and Risley (1995) studied the nature and results of parental interactions with their children as they were acquiring language. The children in the study were members of three levels of socioeconomic status. One group was made up of children of high socioeconomic-level parents, primarily university professors. The second group of children had families who were in the middle-class socioeconomically. The third group children were from families who lived in poverty-level socioeconomic classes.

The study found that parents in all three economic groups interacted with their children in the same basic ways, adjusting their interactive styles as children developed higher levels of skills. However, children living in severe poverty heard far *fewer* words in their interactions at home. They also heard more negative comments and had less encouragement for communication than did children living in more economically advantageous conditions. Several years of observations and follow-up testing demonstrated some important differences in the levels of language skills demonstrated by children in both the middle class and the professional class when compared with children who lived in poverty. The differences in their learning environments were basically quantitative, that is, children living in poverty heard and produced fewer words, had fewer opportunities to interact, and received fewer encouragements to communicate. These differences in environments were reflected in parallel quantitative language deficiencies. Young children of the more economically advantaged families demonstrated larger vocabularies in the observations and tests conducted throughout the studies. In addition, these differences that were demonstrated when children were very young were still present when children were 9 or 10. Thus, it appears that there comes a point when serious differences in the *quantitative* aspects of children's early language experiences are reflected in the overall *quality* of their language. A smaller vocabulary, less experience in talking, and less confidence that talking will be rewarded results in children whose language skills may end up being inadequate for their eventual needs in a competitive and demanding society. It is important to note that the *ability* of these children to learn language is not questioned. The point is that a *child's language environments* have important effects on their language performance.

For these reasons, parent's awareness and their commitment to the ways in which they teach language to their children must be strengthened, particularly among parents struggling in poverty. Such strengthening will take a major effort from professionals in all disciplines, but especially from those in education. Educators working in early childhood education programs are at the forefront of efforts to improve the communication and language learning experiences of their students both at home and in school.

## WHEN SPOKEN WORDS EMERGE, EVERYTHING CHANGES

As typically developing children begin to use spoken words and phrases somewhere between 12 to 18 months, interactions between babies and the other people around them reach still another, higher level. Spoken communicative exchanges occur readily and frequently; the child's world of people becomes, primarily, a verbal one; and this causes previous patterns of interaction to change. For example, when adults were observing babies' actions and "assigning" communicative meaning and significance to them, both parents and children demonstrated a strong tendency to maintain almost constant visual or physical contact with each other. When children begin to use spoken words, however, parents and others are free to ease this need for constant visual monitoring of the child. Instead, adults and children begin to take small steps toward more independence for each. Both begin to trust in the other's availability through communicative messages that do not require them to be in close proximity with one another. Children, for example, learn that the word "mamma," "daddy," or "uh, oh," will usually bring adults to their side. Conversely, parents find that a "call" to their child will evoke a verbal and/or physical response. "Kathy, what are you doing?" might bring a verbal, "Nothing mama," from an out-of-sight Kathy. It is likely, however, that Kathy's mother will seek to confirm this report by moving to a point where she can observe Kathy in her previously out-of-sight location! As spoken communication begins, both adults and children begin a much more intense monitoring of the auditory events that permeate their environment. On hearing the kitchen mixer's motor, children will wander into the kitchen to ask, "What are you making?" Similarly, a loud yell—or in some cases an uncharacteristic lack of any noise at all—will bring mothers or fathers to investigate the circumstances of their child. Parents monitor the speech being used by children at play with one another in another room. By listening to what is being said among playmates, parents can make judgments about the safety of their children's situation.

When their child begins to talk, parents begin to raise their expectations for children's communicative forms. No longer will they respond eagerly to an ambiguous whine or a vague gesture. Instead, the child will begin to hear parents say, "Stop that and tell me what you want" or "Mamma doesn't understand you, tell me." Parents also begin to encourage children to demonstrate their new-found speaking abilities to them and others by exhorting children to, "Tell me what happened in preschool today" or "Tell Grandma what we saw at the store today." "Can you tell the doctor how it feels and where it hurts you?" Although children (and adults) will still use their gestures and body language, more and more these gestures will be accompanied by spoken words and phrases. Thus, much to the delight of both adults and children, it is abundantly clear that children are beginning to be allowed to take their places as functioning members of the full social environment in which they live, play, and learn.

## THE PUSH TO LEARN ACCURATE AND GRAMMATICALLY CORRECT LANGUAGE AND COMMUNICATION SKILLS

When children move fully into the "language community," they are generally welcomed warmly. Parents and grandparents delight in children's often bizarre sentence structures and love to relate the cute sayings that occur daily. Indeed, there is great delight in children's early efforts at using their larger vocabularies and constructing more complex phrases and sentences. Children love being effective in their engagement with the world of people around them. And, in turn, the others around the child like being freed from having to keep the child within their sight, as well as attempting to comprehend their often ambiguous communicative messages conveyed with gestures, tugs, and emotional vocal forms such as cries, squeals, and yelling. However, as soon as the child reaches the level of communication by spoken words, parents, as well as others in the child's world again begin to raise the stakes in the language learning game. Adults who already use language understand that learning one's language is more than learning words and making phrases from these words. Adults know that one must be able to use these abilities to produce language that is:

- *Adequate* for the accurate formulation of messages that the child wants to send to those others around him or her
- *Efficient* in conveying these messages
- *Effective* in getting these communicative messages responded to by receivers

Thus, early language teachers begin to help children refine their language to meet these ideals. Let's look at each of these goals for language use in slightly more detail.

## Adequacy of Language

Because one's language must be capable of encoding and transmitting whatever message a person desires to direct to a receiver, that language system must include a large enough vocabulary to allow a particular message to be expressed. In addition to the vocabulary of words needed for that message, one's language system must reflect a knowledge of the rules by which single words can be strung together to produce the specific *meaning*, or "semantic intentions," that the speaker wishes a partner to receive. These "stringing" rules are carried in what is called the *syntactic* rules of a particular language. Each language has its own particular syntax. In a German, straightforward declarative sentence, for example, the verb most often comes at the end of the sentence. In

English, the verb in a declarative sentence usually will appear in the middle of a sentence, immediately after the subject of the verb and before any object of the verb is stated, for example, "The boy ate the cereal." This verb form and its position in the sentence signal several things about the meaning of the sentence. For example, the action occurred in the past and the boy is the agent of the action of eating. Further, the sentence's syntax indicates that the cereal was the object of the verb and, thus, was the receiver of the boy's act of eating. If we look at a sentence such as, "Is the boy eating cereal?" we see that by putting the auxiliary verb *is* at the front of the sentence and moving the object *cereal* to the final position, we produce a question about the boy's action and the receiver of that action. Another small change in the verb form in this sentence creates a question about a future event: "Is the boy *going* to eat his cereal?"

Mature language users know thousands of variations of vocabulary words. They understand that they can use "grammatical markers," such as adding different endings on verbs and nouns, *go-going* or *boy-boys*. In addition, they know the rules for variations in word orders that change the meaning in sentences such as those we showed above. All of this knowledge about language allows speakers of a language to *mean* just about anything that they want to mean in an utterance. This is why people's vocabularies continue to grow throughout life. It is also why they learn specialized vocabularies and syntactic forms that are specific to their specialized knowledge, interests, and careers.

Mature language users also know that it is easier to *mean* some things than others. For example, most of us use many foreign words and phrases for meanings that can be expressed more easily in another language than in English. Rather than use English, we have found that saying, *"Deja vu"* is an easy and efficient way of indicating an event that has just been experienced but seems to have been experienced at some previous time. As we have mentioned, members of the French culture object strenuously to the reverse option of using American words in their conversations. It is, however, a difficult stance for them to maintain. How else could they refer accurately to, *"le Big Mac "*?

The point of this discussion is simply to note that children begin to use language with only a smidgen of the semantic (meanings) and syntactic knowledge that they need to be able to construct all of the messages that they might need to produce as they grow older. Again this is another reason why we teach much of our language to young children in the context of their interactions with their parents, siblings, and others. It is within these interactions that we can figure out what children want and need to say and help them to acquire needed words and the ways for putting these words together in order to convey their intended meanings. So, we are always gently correcting first the *content* and then the *forms* of children's utterances. When it is necessary to make their utterances more accurately carry their intended message, we provide models of the new words and syntactic forms they might need to produce the specific meaning they intend. Throughout this process we are regularly amazed and amused by some of the things that children say as they struggle to learn the words and the language rules that are required to mean what they want to mean. We suffer slight embarrassments as they learn that all men are not "daddy" and we cringe a bit as we hear them say such things as, "I gots two penny." When errors in conveying accurate meaning in the correct form occur, parents and other mature language users who have frequent contacts with young children often ignore the errors if the child has succeeded in expressing his or her meaning adequately. If the accuracy or the grammar of the utterance is more serious, however, they have two major strategies for helping young children acquire effective language: they *emend* and *expand* children's utterances.

## Emending

The term *emending* is used to identify certain kinds of acts that parents use when they *correct* children's utterances. A specialized word is used to label this strategy because it is a special kind of correction. Emending is, most often, rather indirect and nonconfrontational. For example, if a child says, "I gots two penny," when he has three pennies, a parent will usually do two things— usually with a single response. First, he or she will confirm the "truth value" of the child's utterance and, then, will offer a correction of the utterance and utter the message in more correct grammatical form: "No, you've got three pennies." Second, a parent may also add a model of the correct utterance, "Now you say it, I've got three pennies." We should note that adults don't emend *all* of the incorrect utterances of young children. Rather, they pick those that they feel the child is ready and able to manage or those that are truly important in terms of meaning.

### Expanding

This is a special form of correcting a child's utterance. It involves the modeling of an expanded form of the child's utterance by an adult. The modeled utterance is more complete and, therefore, more correct. In this way, a parent offers the child exposure to the next higher level of grammar that he or she will need. For example, a child might say, "Horsie run," and a parent will say, "Yes, the horsie is running. The horsie is running fast." A child says, "Daddy, bye-bye," and a daycare provider might say, "Yes, Daddy has gone bye-bye. He went to his office to work." In our earlier example of a child's phrase, "I gots two penny," an adult might also say, "No, you've *got* three pennies. One penny, two pennies, three pennies." In this way the adult not only corrects accuracy of the child's utterance but also provides a highly salient contrast between the singular form *penny* and the plural form *pennies.*

These two strategies, emending and expanding children's utterances, are extremely effective because the adult takes the message that the child understands and intends to send, confirms and accepts it— and then offers a better version back to the child. This, you can see, is the epitome of teaching language to children that is "here and now." The adult is actually teaching the correct way to say and mean what the *child* wants to say and mean. Very often, in these cases of emending or expanding, children will imitate the adult's modeled utterance and receive even more approval from the adult. In Chapter 4 when we look at the specific strategies reflected in children's efforts to learn language, we will discuss how children focus on and use these adult corrections both to learn what to say and to better comprehend what certain words, grammatical markers, and word orders truly mean. Grammatical markers, as we have indicated previously, are words and parts of words that indicate functions that are required by a particular language's grammar rules, for example, plural markers for nouns and past tense markers for verbs.

Throughout this period of teaching more of the specifics of the language system, parents and other adults show a rather remarkable ability to keep their language modeling and correction activities just beyond the current level of the child's language skills. That is, the complexity and sophistication of adult language to children tends to be just a bit in advance of the child's. This assures that the child can readily comprehend the adult's language and that there are things that he or she can learn from it. Parents and other adults constantly adjust their language levels to maintain this gap. In this way, adults are always making the child stretch his or her own language skills just a bit further. During this period, too, parents and other adults maintain the practice of keeping their speech relatively slow, well-articulated, and simple but grammatically correct. Table 3–1 summarizes the key adult strategies for language teaching that we have discussed in this chapter.

In the later stages of early childhood, parents and other caregivers begin to get help from formal schooling as teachers weigh

### Table 3–1

Adult Strategies for Facilitating the Communication and Language Learning of Young Children

---

- Respond whenever possible to the apparent intent of a child's physical, facial, vocal, gestural, or language behaviors

- Talk to the child frequently about things that are "here and now" and mark the segments of events that the child is seeing, feeling, and/or hearing

- Modify your normal speech and language in the following ways:

    Use short utterances

    Use complete, but simple sentences

    Use proper grammar, but use vocabulary words that the child can understand

    Repeat a message frequently and paraphrase it if the child seems not to understand it

    Slow down normal speech rate and slightly exaggerate vocal intonation and stress

    Enunciate words clearly

    Emend child utterances

    Expand child utterances

    Adjust language level so that it is just beyond the child's current level

---

in for the indomitable task of helping our children to attain language proficiency and adequacy. Vocabulary learning is stressed and the correct grammar of a culture's language is modeled and formally presented to children beginning in kindergarten and continuing on through the full range of a child's educational experience. People simply must be able to *mean* what they want to *mean* and need to be able to communicate their meanings effectively to others. An adequate vocabulary and a grammatically correct language system are the keys to being able to do so.

## Efficiency of Language

There is another rule that we follow as we converse with other people, and that rule states that we should not impose on another person's time and goodwill unnecessarily. Simply put, this rule states that we should be *efficient* in our communicative interactions. Children are not born understanding this rule. All of us have suffered through a child's long, meandering description of a movie or television show that he or she has seen. The narrative goes on and on. As listeners, we become more and more impatient to end the discussion. It has been said that most children are natural *filibusterers*. Clearly, children sometimes become enamored of their power to use language and they may seek to maintain a listener's attention by talking on and on and on. This is the point in a child's development when one will often hear a parent joke, "I worked so hard to teach him to talk. Now, how do I shut him up"?

Of course, one of the other factors at work in these filibusters is that young children might not yet trust their language skills and, thus, may engage in providing more and more language to ensure that their message is adequate to communicate what they desire to communicate. As children begin to trust that their language skills are adequate to say what they want to say, the need for these long dialogues diminishes. In addition, as children become confident that their listeners are responsive to their communicative efforts, their need to overload the system lessens. Children also learn that caregivers can become impatient with them if their needs for attention become overly demanding. The role of parents and others in the environment, then, is to be responsive to children's communicative efforts and, again, to continue to work on the ability of children to mean what they want to mean—*efficiently.*

It's a fine line that children's listeners must walk. However, experience of both children and their communicative partners usually brings about a balance between being appropriately responsive to children's efforts, while still letting them know when they are breaking the rules of good conversation. In other words, children discover the rules of the conversation game by learning to be both *efficient* and *effective* with their language.

## Effectiveness of Language

There is one more aspect of language that children must be taught and this relates to the rules for using language in ways that increase the probability that their utterances will be responded to adequately and appropriately. Cultures have rules for language use: there is a right way to talk to people and a wrong way. These rules can all be grouped under the general rubric of *politeness*. However, there are many, many ways that the appropriate degree of politeness is achieved. In Chapter 1, we made the point that people have several languages. That is, they talk to different people or audiences in different ways. They use different word choices with certain people. They even use different phrase and sentence structures with one person and not others. These differences result from a speaker's judgment about the degree of politeness needed when talking with others. The degree of politeness needed is determined by the speaker's judgment about his or her relative social relationship with his or her listener. We pointed out that people generally speak to a worker who is subordinate to them in a manner that is different from that used with a friend. In turn, people speak to their bosses differently than they do to their close friends.

### The Concept of Register

The differences between the levels and degrees of politeness and formality of a person's language style are referred to in the psycholinguistic literature as *the register* of one's language in a particular conversational context (Lakoff, 1977). In lay terms, we often refer to it as the *tone of someone's utterances.*

Quite obviously, the relative appropriateness of one's *register* has a great deal to do with the response that his or her utterance receives from a conversational partner. If the register is too "familiar" in tone, it might not receive the best response from a boss, a teacher, or, if the speaker is a young child, a parent or grandparent. Early on, children's language *registers* are often inappropriate, and care is taken by parents and other caregivers and teachers to teach them to begin to modulate the relative politeness of their language to others:

"We don't say, 'hey you,' to your teacher."

"Don't talk that way to grandma, be polite."

"If you ask me again in a nicer way, I'll give you a cookie."

"Don't get sassy with me, young man."

Even with their many lapses, however, by age 4 most young children begin to show an awareness of this notion of *register* and begin to reflect differential degrees of politeness to adults and to children younger than themselves. Often, however, they reflect their knowledge of the differences in language styles by reserving a repertoire of less-than-polite terms to be addressed to their peers. There seems to be some real fun in breaking the rules, such as calling a good pal *boogerhead*.

As they mature, children gradually acquire a full complement of *registers* that will allow them to operate on a world of different people with some effectiveness. They might even begin to reflect an adult style of using what are called "indirect directives." Thus, instead of "I want dinner, Mom," we might hear, "Mom, I'm hungry," or even "Is anyone else hungry besides me"?

As professionals, you know that language learning is a lifetime endeavor. We never stop learning new vocabulary, new registers, and new phrases. Often, we even learn to express all of our world knowledge in languages that are different from our native tongue. If we reflect a bit on our knowledge and experience, we will recall the often-heard observation that the best way to learn a language is to live in the culture in which it is used. Our children do just this as they learn their first language. As we have tried to make evident in this chapter, people within their language culture are working mightily to help them do so from the moment they are born.

## REVIEW: THE ADULTS' ROLE IN THE TEACHING OF BASIC PEOPLE AND THING SKILLS TO CHILDREN

This chapter began with the point that children are *taught* communication by all of the people in their environment. It is the child's primary caregivers—usually mothers—who spend the most time and effort in this teaching endeavor. Obviously, however, fathers, siblings, grandparents, neighbors, and daycare providers are also heavily involved in this process. In fact, it is a rather basic commitment of all of the language-using people in a culture to help their children acquire the culture's primary language system.

In this chapter and the one before it, we provided the details of the kinds of strategies that parents and other adults and children, who already know and use their culture's language, follow in helping to facilitate a young child's discovery and learning of the rudiments of "people skills": the social interaction patterns, communication, and language that will allow him or her to interact successfully and productively with other people. We also discussed the fact that, in this period of early childhood, adults and other children have a parallel set of strategies for introducing children to the rudiments of the basic "thing skills" that they will need to operate on the things of their physical world.

In these chapters we stressed that both the sensorimotor knowledge and communication and language is learned by doing, that is, these skills are first taught in the context of children's interactions with both people and things. Therefore, adult strategies for helping children to discover both thing skills and people skills are applied in contexts in which children and adults are involved in activities in which they are actually *doing something*. They are engaged in cooperative activities that allow each of them a role and further require each of them be responsive to the other. All cultures have strategies for setting up these interactive contexts, although they vary somewhat both between and within cultures. In most Western cultures, interactive contexts in which children and their partners are engaged in productive activities are usually readily available. Parents and other caregivers make sure that they are so that *interactive contexts* are available for language teaching.

Full participation in their overall environment, requires that children must have learned how to interact both with people *and* with the physical elements of their environment. Consequently, they must learn the skills necessary to do so. As we have learned from research and have emphasized in this book, children learn these skills primarily from knowledgeable adults. Adults set out to help children learn the most basic skills that they will need to participate in the interactive contexts in which they will learn language and many other life skills. Some of the more prominent adult strategies for facilitating language learning are summarized in Table 3–1.

Most of the teaching strategies we have identified come instinctively and naturally to most adults. Obviously, however, carrying out this overall pattern of teaching is easier for some people than for others. Such teaching is demanding and time consuming. In many situations it calls for patience and good humor that might be missing at times in a stressful and demanding life. In some cases, people's life circumstances might work against their having the time, energy, or other resources to carry out this teaching demand. It is important to remember, however, that in most of life's important learning, the teaching process is a bit overdesigned. This means that parents and others in the child's environment can *fail to be perfect* and yet still be successful in preparing a child with the language and knowledge skills needed to be successful in life. It is also true, however, that if the significant adults in a child's world truly neglect this teaching requirement their child's learning will be negatively effected.

Breakdowns in this teaching-learning process also can occur because of a child-centered problem rather than a failure by the adults in a child's world. We know that there are physical, emotional, and mental disabilities among children that can prevent them from fully utilizing the teaching provided by caring adults. In the final chapter of this book, we will look at potential breakdowns in both the teaching and the learning processes. We will discuss the possible remedial or compensatory actions that might be taken in these cases.

This chapter focused on the efforts that parents and other adults and children make to help young babies to learn to communicate and to acquire their culture's language system. Now, we need to become more aware of the child's role in this teaching-learning process. Children work hard at learning in all domains. However, because the adults around them emphasize language so much, and because children discover the power of communication and language so early in their lives, they give extraordinary efforts to this particular learning task. Children have their own set of special techniques for utilizing the experiences that adults make available to them. In the following chapter, we will discuss children's contributions to this important effort.

## SUMMARY

- Children are taught communication by all the people in their environment. It is the basic commitment of all of the language-using people in a culture to help their children acquire the cultures primary language system.

- Parents, other adults, and other children who already know their culture's language use a variety of strategies to help a young child learn the social interaction patterns, communication, and language that will allow him or her to interact successfully and productively with other people.

- When young children begin using their language, their communicative partners begin to raise the stakes to demand more language, as opposed to gesture, in the communicative interaction.

- Parents and other adults emend and expand the children's utterances to provide a model of a more accurate or complete version of what the child said. This exposes children to the next level of grammar that will be needed.

- Children learn how to be efficient communicators by observing and learning from the responses of their communicative partners. Parents and others will let children know when they have imposed too much on the listeners attention span.

- Parents and adults teach children the rules for using language most effectively to bring about desired effects on other people in different situations. This includes the abstract, but ever so important, concept of politeness.

## References

Hart, B., & Risley, T. R. (1995). *Meaningful differences in the everyday experience of young American children.* Baltimore: Paul H. Brookes.

Lakoff, R. (1977). *What can you do with words: Politeness, pragmatics, and performatives.* Paper presented at the Texas conference on Performatives, presuppositions, and implicatures, Arlington, TX.

Nelson, K. (1973). Structure and strategy in learning to talk. *Monographs of the Society for Research in Child Development, 38*(149).

# 4

# CHILDREN'S ACTIVE ROLE IN THEIR LEARNING OF COMMUNICATION AND LANGUAGE

## JAMES McLEAN

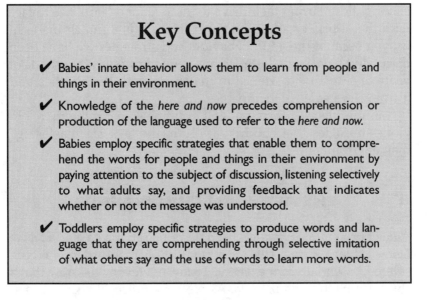

## Key Concepts

✔ Babies' innate behavior allows them to learn from people and things in their environment.

✔ Knowledge of the *here and now* precedes comprehension or production of the language used to refer to the *here and now*.

✔ Babies employ specific strategies that enable them to comprehend the words for people and things in their environment by paying attention to the subject of discussion, listening selectively to what adults say, and providing feedback that indicates whether or not the message was understood.

✔ Toddlers employ specific strategies to produce words and language that they are comprehending through selective imitation of what others say and the use of words to learn more words.

## INTRODUCTION

In the last chapter, we discussed the many ways that parents and other people in a young child's environment help their babies learn about the world of people and things in which they live. As you have seen, it is an all-out and demanding effort for parents and others in the child's environment.

Research has shown that typically developing young children have a strong motivation to master their environment (White, 1959; Yarrow, Morgan, Jennings, Harmon, & Gaiter, 1982). Included in this "mastery motivation" that Yarrow and others described are drives to discover and learn about both the social and physical world. In the social domain, interaction skills and patterns, nonlinguistic communicative skills, and spoken language are the major skills to master. Fortunately, very young babies have a strong drive to join into the social environment that surrounds them. Thus, they learn to interact actively and cooperatively with the people around them. They first work diligently to understand the language that is so pervasive in their environment and, then, to learn to produce this powerful and useful behavior themselves.

A physical world of things also surrounds infants and, like the social world, offers them a nearly infinite source of stimulation and learning. In such a rich, dual environment of experiences, children bring their drive to discover and learn face to face with the efforts of adults to teach them. It is a match made in heaven because the adult behaviors and strategies we have been discussing have been designed and refined through thousands of years of human experience to match up with the abilities and learning strategies of their babies.

In this chapter, then, we will examine some of the more obvious strategies that children apply in the task of "mastering" their environment.

## THE NEWBORN CHILD'S MIND

A newborn child's *mind* has been described in the past as a *tabula rasa*—a "blank slate." This meant that, at birth, the mind was considered, essentially, nonexistent. Today, however, we know that a child begins to learn *in utero*. As we have noted in previous discussion, before they are born, babies learn to recognize their mother's voice and discriminate it from all other voices in their environment. We know, too, that babies are able to make some discriminations of their culture's speech sounds from those of other languages. Before a child is born, millions of the neurons in his or her brain have already been "wired" to perform the basic physiological functions that sustain a baby's life. These so called *autonomic systems* of the brain control such bodily functions as heart activity, body temperature control, and the regulation of glandular productions. A child's brain is also constructed so that, even before birth, the senses of hearing, touch, and body-position awareness (proprioception) have already received incoming stimuli from the outside world. Babies' senses of sight, respiration, and smell and taste are also "prewired" to function, in at least rudimentary fashion, at birth.

Since early in their *in-utero* developmental phases, preborns have probably received millions of bits of auditory stimuli, including human speech, both from mother and from outside sources. Prior to birth children have also experienced *proprioceptive stimuli*, which include sensory feelings associated with bodily movements and changing pressures on the body. The most basic neurological reflexes are intact before birth, so babies "startle" and kick under certain conditions of stimulation. Preborns can probably sense heat and cold as well and perhaps, pain, although certain chemicals in a mother's body function to prevent some pain sensations. The point is that, at birth, typically developing children have brains that have already functioned for several months to sustain certain of their bodily functions and to allow them opportunities to experience some of the sensory stimuli of the world they are about to enter. At birth, then, that brain and its potential for millions of connections between its neurons is literally starved for additional stimulation and is ready to begin to form those connections that reflect what we call *learning*.

## THE MECHANICS OF LEARNING

As you no doubt already know, the brain operates on the basis of electrical impulses that travel along networks of neurons. Certain chemicals in the brain enhance the conduction of these impulses and help them to move along the neural pathways by crossing the small gaps between the ends of its neurons. These currents in the brain are created when the brain receives a *stimulus*. Many stimuli to the brain are electrical events that are sent there by the receptors of the body's five senses. Thus, everything a baby sees, hears , smells, tastes, or feels creates neural connections in a part of the brain specifically designated to receive information from each of these senses. If an event triggers several of these senses simultaneously, each of the various sensual stimuli is received by a different part of the brain. Connections *within* these sections of the brain are created and, in addition, connections are also made *between* the different brain areas involved. The more times that the same event occurs, the smaller the gaps between the neurons along certain pathways in the brain become. Pathways with smaller gaps between neurons are easier for brain impulses to cross and, thus, are more easily traveled by stimuli. The more easily stimuli can travel, the stronger the pathways become. The stronger pathways become, the more easily the experiences that created these pathways can be "recalled" by the infant. For example, as young infants nurse, they have a visual stimulus of their mother. They also experience smell and taste stimuli from the event. They hear the mother's voice and her speech. They experience the ways she holds and caresses them. All of these experiences are received by different parts of the brain where they are associated with the several other stimuli received at the same time by other parts of the brain. After this event has been experienced hundreds of times, the pathways for it are well established among the neurons of the brain, and the child's *mind* now contains a basic concept of an event that can be discriminated from all the others that he or she experiences.

When several of the same stimuli are received in contexts other than feeding, existing concepts are revised and expanded. For example, the visual, auditory, and olfactory stimuli associated with *mother* will be separated from the feeding experience and babies will come to "know" that mother exists as an entity separate both from themselves and from the feeding event. This reception, cataloging, and association of millions of incoming stimuli that create the neural pathways that, in turn, *creates learning*.

Despite all that babies have learned before they are born, millions of neurons in the baby's brain are still waiting to be stimulated and shaped into a *mind*. The bulk of this *mind-shaping* learning does not occur until they enter the outside world of people and things that make up the environment in which they will live. At this point the typically developing infant's brain already reflects some learning and is poised and ready to begin to receive more and more information from the world. The infant will then catalogue it, associate it with other information received, store it away for recall, and thus have it available for connecting it to past and future experiences. Beginning with just a little information, newborn infants make up for lost time as they begin to receive and process every scrap of visual, auditory, proprioceptive, olfactory, and touch stimuli that they experience. Every noise, every sight, every smell, every movement and touch stimulates their brain and is perceived and stored. Thus, as noted in the example above, children very quickly learn to visually recognize *mother* and to discriminate her (and her voice) from all other persons. They learn to recognize *daddy* and their siblings in the social environment around them. They learn to associate certain sounds with the events that produce them (e.g., "Someone is entering my space"). Certain odors mean "food." Certain textures and odors mean a favorite blanket or stuffed toy. The touch sensation created by a finger or small rattle being placed in the baby's hand will evoke a "grasping" reflex that allows babies to hold and move objects. Certain sounds, such as those from a familiar person or a frequently present music box, come to bring comfort to an anxious infant. Hunger evokes fussing and crying. Previously unknown sounds may evoke fear or discomfort in a baby. Similarly, people who are strangers in a baby's regular environment also can evoke negative reactions. Being cuddled by a well-known person, however, brings about the recall of previous, pleasant events and, thus, is soothing. Very quickly then, the *tabula* isn't so *rasa* anymore and the learning explosion is on—never to stop during a lifetime.

In the next chapter, we will look in more detail at the specifics of children's early learning of some very basic people and thing skills. In this chapter, however, we want to discuss the special ways that children behave in order to learn what they want and need to learn. As with most activities and processes in these early developmental stages, typical children seem to reflect certain *universal* behavioral tendencies—tendencies that work remarkably well in helping them to extract information from the environment of both people and things. It is this information, then, that allows them to learn the crucial information and skills that they will need both to live in their developmental world, and, later, to gain the additional, complex knowledge they will need to successfully negotiate the challenges of their individual and unique lifetime.

## Matching Adult Teaching Strategies and Infant Learning Strategies

When we talk about a baby's learning strategies in these early stages of development, we don't mean that the behaviors that we will be discussing are consciously planned by babies. We simply mean that a number of outside influences, including the particular interactive and teaching strategies of adults we discussed in the preceding chapter, interact with certain behavioral characteristics of babies and their active brains to create certain consistent patterns of behaviors—patterns that become stable and are repeated by babies. Children's behavioral repertoires reflect many such tendencies or "strategies" that allow them to be successful in creating the events that produce the stimuli needed to learn about many different aspects of their world. It might seem a bit obtuse to talk about "creating events that produce the stimuli needed to learn," but we must always remember that knowledge and learning are the products of individuals' *discoveries* derived from their own experiences. The often-heard admonition that we must always learn things the "hard way" recognizes the fact that we most often must experience something ourselves in order to really learn about it. This need to experience and discover for ourselves leads to some of the greatest frustrations of parenthood as we try to tell our children certain truths, only to have them ignore us and proceed to find those truths for themselves—too often, "the hard way."

As we will see, the strategies reflected in very young children's learning behaviors and the strategies reflected in adult teaching behaviors complement one another. In fact, in many cases, they seem to be near reciprocals of one another. For example, adults tend to exaggerate and repeat key words in their utterances and children tend to focus on these key words in their parents' utterances. This suggests, of course, that these child and adult strategies allow parents and children to influence one another. In fact, as we look at both of them in more detail in this chapter, we will see this mutual influence rather clearly. It is obvious that, early on, the adults' strategies necessarily lead the way in these teaching-learning interactions. But babies' reactions and their relative success or failure in discovering what adults intend for them to experience and learn can either reinforce the adult strategies or cause them to be revised or discarded.

## A BRIEF REVIEW OF ADULT STRATEGIES

You will recall from our discussions in Chapter 2 that adult strategies for helping children discover important things about the world are many and varied. First, they engage the infant in interactions that involve both activities with the physical world and the social world of people. They make sure that they share a "common focus" with the child. They flood the child with language and other auditory stimulation such as rattles, squeaky toys, music boxes, and music. They also provide infants with objects to feel, see, and manipulate. They practice turn taking and provide interactive games such as peek-a-boo and "find the rattle" being hidden behind the adult's back. They simplify their language input to the child by using simple sentences and phrases and talking slowly and emphasizing key words. They paraphrase their messages a lot and they repeat key words and phrases. They leave gaps in their interactions to provide infants with opportunities to respond. They teach infants to do things with objects and toys (e.g., shake rattles, hug teddy bears, and roll balls). A look at the commercial baby toys that permeate a typical child's environment reveals a huge collection of busy boxes, stackable materials, pull toys, and inviting containers for receiving objects. Clearly, the toy designers have read the child development data and are ready to help the adults provide infants with a wealth of sensory experiences and socially interactive episodes that stimulate, and thus, "program" the neurons of their brain and to create the pathways that constitute discovery or learning.

As we review these adult strategies for providing children a rich world of sensory stimuli and social experience, it seems clear that they are sincere and clear efforts to facilitate infant learning. Thus, we have come to call this constellation of adult activities—"learning facilitation strategies" (Snyder & McLean , 1977).

## INFANT STRATEGIES FOR GAINING KNOWLEDGE ABOUT THE PEOPLE AND THINGS IN THEIR ENVIRONMENT

In response to adult efforts to facilitate their experience and discovery, children's behaviors begin to reflect tendencies that allow them to use these adult-provided experiences effectively. The infant has much to experience and discover. We have noted that an infant has a tremendous motivation and drive to master his or her environment. It is important for us to appreciate the complexity of the environment that the newborn child faces. First, it is a world of almost endless stimulation of all his or her senses. There are thousands of things to see, hear, touch, smell, and taste. There are also thousands of instances where there are internal feelings to experience—hunger, physical discomfort, movement, pain, and even sneezing. There are interactive sensations to experience and catalogue—snuggling, feeding, being carried from place to place, and being left alone. Faced with all of these stimuli and sensations and with a brain that fairly cries out for stimulation, an infant clearly must work diligently to experience this world and impose some order and sense to it. This work to learn can be better appreciated if we look more carefully at the behavioral tendencies or "strategies" that have been identified in babies' earliest interactions with their worlds (Snyder & McLean, 1977; Snyder-McLean & McLean, 1978). Let's look at three basic types of these early learning strategies:

1. Attend to, and act on, the environment;

2. Actively observe, listen and learn from other people; and

3. Explore and experiment.

### Infant General Learning Strategy 1: Attend to and Act on the People and Objects in the Environment

Have you ever been seated next to a couple with an infant in a restaurant? You glance at the infant and see that she is looking at you—watching your every move. After you smile, wave, and say "Hi" to her, you are aware that the baby is watching you handle your eating utensils, bring food to your mouth, chew, and drink. To be sure, it is a bit disconcerting—but you know that it is all a part of the baby's game—and in between smiles at the baby and her parents, you continue your eating routine. Hopefully, someone will soon occupy the table next to you and the baby's attention will shift to another person on whom she can bestow her intense scrutiny. Of course, the new person will wave and say "Hi" and the game will continue. Hopefully, sometime in the next few months, the parents will be instructing the baby that it is "not polite" to watch another person so intently.

Thus, we can be relatively sure that, unless babies are hungry, sleepy, or uncomfortable, they will be almost always in a state of alertness, actively attending to the environment around them. They will most likely be watching, listening, touching, or manipulating the people or objects that surround them. Sometimes they may be practicing making sounds with their vocal tracts and seeing how they might alter these sounds to make other sounds. All parents can recall periods where, after awakening from a nap, their infant would lie in his or her crib and indulge in these long periods of sound production practice called "babbling." At times this babbling practice accompanies an activity in which the baby hits at the elements of the mobile mounted above the crib and intently watches the ensuing action. As the baby's arms flail to strike at the mobile, often, new, louder sounds are emitted. A few days later, long strings of these new sounds emanate from the baby's room, being produced during a long sustained period of flailing away at the mobile. The neuro-connections in the brain have been made and can be recalled; and the behaviors that created these newer, more forceful sounds can be reproduced at will by the infant.

Similarly, people who have observed babies have seen them spend long periods manipulating a set of plastic cups. They grasp them, throw them, taste them, put them into one another, and then throw them again. How many times have you had a baby on your lap remove your glasses from your head, then put them back on your head, then take them off again, and on and on the game is played.

We previously noted how quickly children learn to take turns when afforded an opening to do so. We know, too, that very young children soon *initiate* turn-taking games with adults.

Thus, babies are constantly replaying things that they have learned. As they observe and act on their environment, they are creating new pathways among the neurons of their brain. With this new learning, they are also combining and modifying older pathways so that their minds are gradually, but quickly, being expanded and their existing knowledge holdings are refined. So, in addition to learning new things, babies are also extremely happy to repeat previously learned activities. Favorite toys are established as babies learn what actions on certain toys bring them the most interesting results. They are, in other words, happy to be competent in their play with familiar toys. They love "peek-a-boo" because they have learned how to play this particular game. For the same reason, infants love to look at the same books over and over again. They are also happiest in their own beds—with their favorite blanket, teddy bear, and music box.

In a remarkably short time, then, infants have established many millions of connections in their brains and have begun to develop their own unique minds. Their individual minds reflect the sum of all of their previous experiences and the learning that has resulted from these experiences.

## Infant General Learning Strategy 2: Observe , Listen, and Learn From Other People

At a few months of age, infants have made the connection that other people around them are a primary source for knowledge about how and what to do to master their environment. They have, for example, been highly rewarded for doing what mother or daddy does. Thus, when they take turns they have learned to observe the adult's demonstration of the action called for in a particular situation and have done their best to reproduce the adult's actions in that situation. If their reproduction is not quite right, they have discovered that mother or father will take their hands and directly help them perform the correct motor act. In learning from others in their environment, then, children take *instruction* from them.

### Imitation

In their first few months children can only imitate actions that they can see themselves produce. Thus, they can imitate an adult reach or grasp. They can watch both themselves and mother in a mirror and match actions. Around 7 months or so, however, most children can imitate actions without being able to see themselves. They have gained enough *proprioceptive* experience to know, at least roughly, what position their limbs are in and what changes need to be made to approximate the actions of their imitative model. To be sure, some of these imitations are only approximations of an adult's actions because infants of this age do not yet have fine motor movements in all of their extremities. For example, they might experience difficulty in letting go of an object. Thus, most parents know that the first acts of "giving" mother an object might be more of a throw than a give. Parents are sensitive to such limitations in children's abilities, however, and they accept imitations that are even close to their model.

In the second 6 months of children's lives, they begin to reflect all kinds of abilities to carry out the appropriate actions with many items in their environment. They take mother's hat and put it on their head. They put daddy's glasses on their heads. They take spoons and "stir" in pots and pans. They put mother's necklace around their neck. Thus, in addition to being able to imitate actions that they cannot see themselves carry out, they are also reflecting all of the knowledge that their active attending has allowed them to discover. They bang drums, hit things with hammers, and feed their dolls with minature bottles. Clearly, typical infants approaching their first birthday have learned many of their behaviors from watching and imitating those around them. They are, essentially, doing what other people do. They belong to, and in, the world of both people and things.

### Seeking and Taking Instructions

There is a natural extension of the general imitation tendencies of very young children. This tendency is to look to adults (or other children around them) for instructions in behaviors they have not yet mastered. Thus, a frequent activity for a young child is to take a toy and hand it to another person. The intention that adults assign to such an act is, "Show me what to do with this—show me how it works." At other times, babies might attempt to open a jar or make a music box play without success. After such a failure, an infant will often look at an adult and then look back at the toy; or perhaps he or she will attempt the task again and then look at the adult. In these cases the infant seems to be saying, "See, I really tried, but I need help." In most cases, the adult is ready to help the baby open the jar or wind up the music box—either directly or by taking the baby's hands and putting them through the needed action. Note that, in such episodes, the child's request is "sincere" in that she has tried and failed. Similarly, adults follow the rules for human interactions by responding to the child's communicative act in a sincere and constructive manner.

In such helpful teaching episodes, adults often help a child learn by, as Jerome Bruner (Bruner 1975) has described, "scaffolding" for them on a task. In scaffolding, or "reverse-chaining," an adult sets up situations so that a child only has to do only a small action to complete a task. In an earlier example, we described how an adult might turn the handle on a jack-in-the-box up to the point where only one more turn of the handle will cause the clown to pop up, then will put the baby's hand on the handle and let the baby make the last small turn of the handle to be successful in attaining the clown's popping out of the box. Similarly, an adult might unscrew a jar lid until it is almost off and then help the child make that last, small unscrewing movement and take off the lid. The next time these tasks occur, the adult will complete a bit less of the required task and allow the child to do more. In this way, adults teach children how to do these things, but they arrange the task so that children can experience some immediate success, see what the end result of the "chain" is, and not become frustrated by having to do more of the task than they can handle at any given time.

## Infant General Learning Strategy 3: Explore and Experiment!

In addition to interactions to seek and accept help from adults and other children around them, babies spend long periods of time acting on objects in isolation. They will, for example, play with their blocks, plastic cups, or toy mailboxes for hours—experimenting and learning how to stack and put things inside one another. Each action and each success is recorded in the brain and is maintained there as an established pathway that is combined with past learning. Of course, a lot of early learning will be need to revised as later experiences add new material to the child's knowledge base.

Besides physically acting on objects, we have already noted that infants also watch and listen intently. As they near the three-quarter mark of their first year, infants have stored up thousands of bits of information through observation. This observational learning coupled with "learning by doing" means that an alert, active infant has piled up millions of pathways in the neurons of his or her brain. The baby has a grand storehouse of knowledge about both the objects and the people in his or her environment. We will detail this knowledge in Chapter 5. At this point, however, we want to introduce you to a second set of tendencies that children's behaviors reflect: strategies that they apply specifically to learning the spoken language of their environment.

## INFANTS' LANGUAGE COMPREHENSION LEARNING STRATEGIES

### Knowledge About the World Must Come Before Language

We have discussed children's early learning about the people and things of their environment. We studied this before concentrating on their strategies for learning language for a very important reason. As we have stressed, children must have a good store of knowledge about people and things *before* they can learn language. The reason this knowledge is necessary is because language itself *refers to* the people, things, actions, and happenings in the environment. When people use language, they use it to talk (or write or read) about things that they know about the world in which they live, work, and play. People use language to have effects on other people and they can do this only if they refer to things that they, *and* their listeners, know about. Lois Bloom, a researcher in child language development was among the first to point out that a child's language "maps onto" his or her *existing knowledge* (Bloom, 1970). In a sense, then, people simply cannot talk about something that doesn't exist in their knowledge base. Similarly, if we use language to refer to something about which our listener has no knowledge, the message simply isn't understood. Basically, then, when we talk about a person, a thing, or an event we are using symbols that *refer* to those topics to evoke our listeners' knowledge about those persons, things, or events. Thus, until a baby knows something about people, things, or events, he or she cannot learn to comprehend or produce the language by which they can refer to these things.

## The First *Language Learning* Task: Learn How to Comprehend What Words Mean (Refer to)

If young children are to learn to comprehend and produce language, they must first learn to connect the words and phrases that they hear to the people, things, events, and/or states to which a speaker is referring. Thus, a baby must first figure out what an adult is trying to *mean* in his or her message and then figure out the relationships between the words adults use and the meanings they intend. This task might seem like a "Catch 22" before we explore it a bit. After all, how is a child going to understand what an adult *means* if he or she doesn't understand the words being used? A baby will begin to connect words to real-life people, things, events, and states because of what he or she already knows about the world and because of all of the adult efforts to help the baby connect the right words with the right referent or meaning.

Let us look at a few early examples of how this process works. Children have been playing "peek-a-boo" for months. The routine is well known to them. Each time they play this game, they hear the word "peek-a-boo" uttered at certain times in the action sequence. It does not take long for the child to learn to associate the word with the overall event. Very quickly, he or she learns that the words "peek-a-boo" are always associated with the action of taking one's hands away from his or her eyes. After all, mother, daddy, and sister and brother have demonstrated this relationship many, many times and the baby has seen and heard the actions along with the words. Similarly, he knows that a little furry animal coexists with him in his home. He has been taught how to ". . . pet the *kitty*." To not "hurt the *kitty*." How to ". . . feed the *kitty*." It does not take the baby long to associate the word "kitty" with that furry little entity that roams about in his environment.

In fact, as young children hit their stride in learning words, they often need only *one exposure* to a word to learn it and form a hypothesis about its referent. These examples stress again the importance of the adult strategy of talking about the here and now, the items that are present, or the actions that are occurring at the time of the interaction with a young child. We have noted that interactions must take place around an item or event on which both the child and the adult are focused. When children recognize and share the *common focus* of the interaction and the language being used in it, they have taken the first step at discovering the connection between words and phrases and certain objects and events in their environments.

As we review examples of early language learning interactions, we observe that young children typically use *three* very important strategies to help them learn about their language (Snyder & McLean, 1977; Snyder-McLean & McLean, 1978). First, as noted above, we can see that simply attending to the *common focus* of each interaction with another person is an important language-learning strategy for young children. A second strategy that children use in learning to connect words with real life items and events is one we call *selective listening*. Babies who are just beginning to understand words cannot easily discriminate different words from one another. So, they learn to listen carefully to adults, because adults make some words easier to hear by emphasizing them and repeating them. Finally, the third strategy used by young children learning to comprehend language is to behave in ways that provide *feedback* to their adult partners. This feedback tells an adult how well a child comprehended his or her message. We will discuss each of these three strategies more fully in the pages to follow.

## Infant Language Comprehension Strategy 1: Attend to the *Common Focus of an Interaction*

In past discussions we noted that, before adult-child interactions can occur, both partners must adopt a common focus, that is, they must both be attending to and/or interacting with the same object or event. We also noted earlier that, from the very earliest engagements, adult caregivers work very hard to attract and maintain the infant's attention to some person, thing, or event during their interactions. Children learn this lesson rapidly, and almost from the beginning, they focus on the faces and actions of their mothers or the other adults and children around them. They follow their interactive partner's eye-gaze or they focus on the object of the adult's actions. Thus, when babies begin trying to connect the words they hear with the objects and actions that the words refer to, they are already attending to the common focus of the interaction, which is typically the referent for the words they are hearing.

All of these interactions with people and things in the world contribute to the development of the young child's mind. When children are engaged in the common focus of an interaction, their brains are actively processing all of the sights, sounds, and feelings associated with that interaction. This new information is added to information from past experiences already stored in their brains. This growing accumulation of experiences allows children to form and refine both the social and physical world concepts that will be referred to by the words and phrases that they will soon be learning. For example, an infant's first experience with a dog may be simply the sound of the dog barking, heard over the edge of her crib. Thus, her first concept of this event is based just on that sound. Over time, children will add many additional bits of information to their growing concept of "dog-ness": it is furry, it has a cold nose, it licks your face, it runs and jumps and wags its tail, and, at first, it is a brown and black creature that sits on their mother's lap and is called "Rover." Through further experience, this concept will grow to include dogs that are not called Rover, are not brown and black, do not live in their house, and even dogs in picture books. All of his or her experiences with "dogs" are processed and catalogued by the child's developing brain from the moment of birth. So, long before babies learn the words that refer to things and events in their environments, they already have many well-developed concepts about these things and events. In a sense, then, we can say that babies know about the referents of words before they learn to use the words themselves.

Now, let's return to the question of how a baby manages to learn so many words in the first year of life. We can see how the early concepts, or meanings, developed in the baby's mind through his or her earliest experiences, make the language-learning task much less overwhelming. Basically, the baby already knows many entities, actions, and states that language elements will be used to refer to. Thus, the baby only needs to figure out which words go with which referents. Our tendency to speak directly to babies, using exaggerated intonation and stress patterns, and to speak to them about the immediate focus of our interaction further simplifies this learning task. Let's return to our earlier example: mother says, "Nice *kitty*; Can you pet the *kitty*? Yes, pretty *kitty*," just when the baby is attending to the kitty. The baby's active brain is gathering up new information about this experience and mother has made the word *kitty* a very notable part of this experience, ensuring that this word will now be associated with the baby's developing concept of "kittiness."

The same process works for children in learning the meanings for familiar phrases, as well as single words. For example, when looking at a picture book together, a parent might say, "Can you show me the bunny?" Through past experience, the child knows the familiar routine that is being played out and understands that mother or father expects him to look at the book and put his finger on the picture of the bunny. Or, when mother is hugging the doll and hands it to the child, she is expecting the child to match her action on the doll. When she says "Can you *hug* the baby?" the child already knows the action of *hugging*. Thus, when children see that the common focus is one that is familiar to them and they know from experience what action is desired, they can begin to relate the words and phrases that they hear to the familiar actions and routines that they refer to. Remember, mother is emphasizing certain words in her utterance and is repeating them several times as she demonstrates the action, or other response, desired from her child.

By the end of their first year, then, children have become very active participants in their own language learning. We noted earlier that adults do most of the work in establishing joint focus with very young infants. They talk about things the infant is already attending to or produce interesting sounds and movements to attract the child's attention to something that they want to talk about. The older infant, however, is able to share responsibility for finding the common focus of an interaction. The toddler can actively establish a common focus by handing an object to the adult, pointing to some entity or event; or by following the adult's line of visual regard, he or she can easily figure out what the adult is already looking at and talking about.

Thus, as they move into the period of true language learning, children have become full partners in this process and will seek to establish and maintain shared attention with adults and other children in their worlds. With this shared attention established, the child's language learning task is really quite simple: Listen to the adult's *words* and note which items or actions are the common focus in the routine when these words or phrases are spoken. At this point, babies can be engaged in novel routines, ones which they have *not* experienced before, and by following their strategy of identifying the common focus, they can begin to figure out what the words and phrases they are hearing *refer to.* They are learning how to *comprehend* the language around them by connecting the words to the items and actions they are focusing on and experiencing.

### Infant Language Comprehension Strategy 2: Listen Selectively to Adults' Language Input

You already know that adults around very young children produce simple sentences or phrases. They talk slowly, using exaggerated inflections in their voices. They also emphasize the key words in their utterances. They paraphrase and repeat their utterances many times. They establish a *common focus* and talk about things that are "here and now" for the child. Very often, they put the key words at the ends of their sentences and phrases. They are physically oriented toward the child as they talk to him or her. All of these characteristics of adults' talk to children cause the child to "tune in" and to focus on the utterances that they recognize as being directed specifically to them.

When babies tune in to adult utterances and try to connect words they hear to specific aspects of the interactive episode in which they are engaged, they listen selectively to the words that are emphasized and repeated. They tend, then, to ignore many of the "little" words and the unexaggerated words in an incoming utterance. Because very young babies cannot yet discriminate all of the words that adults speak to them, and because they cannot remember all of them in any given sequence, young babies could be overwhelmed by the oceans of words that surround them every day. The adult practice of emphasizing and repeating the key words in their utterances function as life-preservers for them. As a result, the natural tendency of babies to tune in specifically to words that are emphasized, repeated, or occur at the ends of phrases helps them in learning their language. Children have learned to listen *selectively* to adult utterances and to "screen out" less important words in order to focus on the few words that they can handle. Again, we see that an adult strategy to facilitate children's discoveries by highlighting certain words is effective because it is matched by children's selective listening strategies.

## Infant Language Comprehension Strategy 3: Provide Feedback to Adults Regarding Their Messages

We know that children are active in their environments. They observe and listen carefully to incoming stimuli and try diligently to behave appropriately in interactive situations with other people. As adults, we are alert to children's behaviors that reflect their understanding of communication addressed to them. When we talk to young babies, they will usually attend and respond in some way. The babies' responses to communication provide important feedback to their adult partners. Usually, the communication we address to young babies includes many clues to our meaning. In addition to our words, babies get information from our tone of voice, our gestures, our eye gaze, and our facial expressions. Depending on how a child responds, we can infer what meaning he or she has extracted from our communication act. Did the baby correctly understand the overall message of our communication as playful, serious, calming, or angry? Does the response show that he or she understood the specific referent we were talking about? If we said something about our daughter's doll, does her response include looking at or acting on the doll? Did she understand the intent of our communication—whether it was to look at the doll, hug the doll, or give us the doll? The young child's response to communication provides feedback about whether the message of our communicative act was correctly or incorrectly comprehended by the child. In turn, the adult responds to a child's behavior either by rewarding a correct response or gently correcting an inappropriate one.

Because of children's eager readiness to respond to adult attempts at interaction and communication, adults immediately know that a message was not heard or was not understood when a baby *doesn't make an effort to respond*. A child who looks blank and doesn't make a response tells an interacting adult that the message was not heard or was beyond the child's comprehension abilities. Sometimes older babies will simply continue their action in an ongoing interactive routine or activity and ignore a new message that they do not understand. In a sense, children seem to be saying to themselves, "I don't get that last message, so I will simply to continue my last actions to show that I am still *willing* to play." This strategy usually prompts the adult partner to repeat her communication, with additional clues about its meaning. The adult may demonstrate the action she was suggesting ("Look, I am going to *stir* the pudding. Do you want to *stir it*, too?") or add a gesture to indicate the thing she was naming ("OK, you keep the bunny [points to bunny] and I'll play with the *giraffe* [holds up the giraffe]; oh, this *giraffe* is soft; do you want to pet the *giraffe*, too?" [holds out the giraffe]).

We noted earlier that parents, and other mature language users, including older children, use a special language we called "parent-ese" in talking to very young children. One of the remarkable things about this "parent-ese" is that it always seems to be calibrated to just the right level of language complexity for the particular child with whom the adult is interacting. Thus, the same parent will use very different language with a 4-month-old baby than with his 18-month-old sister. Even college sophomores, who don't have a lot of experience with babies, will make these subtle adjustments in their language, depending on the age of the baby they are talking to. At first, this ability of mature language users seems truly amazing. How do we know just what level of language is appropriate for each baby? If you are thinking about the feedback strategies we just discussed, then you already know the answer to this question—babies tell us just what level of language they can manage, by the way they respond to us. It doesn't take long for a baby to train a new communication partner how to talk to her. After all, nobody wants to be ignored when they are trying to communicate—even with a baby!

## INFANT LANGUAGE PRODUCTION STRATEGIES

At about a year of age, give or take a couple of months either way, typically developing babies have acquired a substantial knowledge base about the people and things in their world. They also are having good success at connecting up the language they hear with that knowledge. Children are now ready to move to the next step in their learning of language. They are ready to begin to *produce* language of their own; and adults are more than ready to help in this process! In fact, most of the strategies that adults have been using in the early language comprehension stages are also useful in helping babies of around 1 year in age in learning to produce the words they have learned to comprehend. We know that babies listen *selectively* to adults. That is, they tune in to words and phrases that adults exaggerate, repeat, or place at the end of their utterances. If this strategy is good for helping babies learn to comprehend incoming language—a parallel strategy of *selectively imitating* these particularly salient words and phrases is an equally effective strategy for learning to produce language.

## Infant Production Strategy 1: Imitate Adult Language Selectively

Imagine this scene: 15-month-old Andrew and his mother are walking in the park. Andrew points excitedly at a robin hopping in the grass just ahead of them. His mother looks at the robin and says,: "Oh look at the *birdie*. See the *birdie*. Hop hop hop—*birdie*. Do you see the pretty *birdie*?" How do you expect Andrew to respond to his mother? Most likely, if you have spent any time around toddlers, you can just imagine his response, can't you? He will almost certainly say something like, "Birdie" or "See Birdie" or, because it is at the end of mother's utterance, "Pretty birdie." This simple, familiar type of interaction is played out many times every day in the busy lives of typical toddlers and their caregivers. And, through this type of natural, everyday interaction, typically developing toddlers learn to produce their culture's spoken language. Let's consider how the teaching-learning process worked in the example above.

Adults understand that babies cannot begin their talking by uttering sentences or even long phrases, so they cut up their long language utterances into small, child-size bits. Children listen selectively to this child-sized language and capitalize on the help that they are getting from their teaching partners. At first, babies imitate words that they comprehend. So they learn the names of family members, pets, and the pictures in the books that parents go through with them night after night. They also learn the terms for common actions, such as run, fall-down, and jump, and for various body "states," such as hungry, sleepy, or sick. They also learn the terms for referring to physical world states such as wet, sticky, and hot. We will, of course, look at this early word learning in more detail in the next chapter. For now, it is important to see that the first words children learn and seek out in the early months are those that allow them to refer to people, things, and states in their immediate environment.

Children will also imitate single words and short phrases that are useful for acting on other people, particularly words that actually control other's behaviors—"stop it," "no, mine," "look," "please," "hold me," "give me," "help." Such words and phrases are often offered by parents for their babies to imitate; "Tell Bobby to stop it, tell him . . . *'it's mine.'*" "Ask me nice, say, *'please help mommy.'*" It takes only a few months for infants of 12 to 18 months to acquire a nice vocabulary of words and phrases for conducting all kinds of social business in their little environment. Now it becomes time for them to begin to make their utterances longer and more grammatical. As a result, both young children and parents begin to adjust to these needs to become better language users.

As mentioned previously, parents in these later stages begin to gently correct incorrect utterances. They also begin to demonstrate how to make an utterance longer and more in line with good grammatical usage. In Chapter 3, we labeled these two adult practices as *emending* and *expanding* childrens' utterances. At this stage, parents become less repetitive in their talk to children, and more direct in their corrections of childrens' utterances and their modeling of correct utterance forms.

> **Child:** [While holding out empty cup] "Daddy, juice more"
>
> **Father:** [Looks at child and takes her cup] "More juice?"
>
> **Child:** [Reaches out with empty hand] "More juice!"
>
> **Father:** [Opens juice bottle and starts to pour] "Okay, say, 'please'"
>
> **Child:** "More juice, please" [Takes cup filled with juice]

Children at this stage will selectively imitate whole phrases or the corrected parts of phrases that adults have emended or expanded for them. Children want to learn how to do this magical thing called talking, and adults are anxious for them to become competent talkers. There is little doubt that using language makes life much easier for both children and adults. It allows them to communicate more efficiently and to interact, through their spoken communication, even when they are out of each other's sight.

## Infant Production Strategy 2: Using Language to Learn Language

My oldest son seems to have been born talking. However, my younger son, blessed (or cursed) with an older brother who did most of the talking for both of them, was a bit slower in acquiring an adequate oral language repertoire. He has since more than made up for this slight delay— but I will always remember his, "What's that stuff what" strategy for learning language. For example, "Daddy" ("What Tommy?") "What's that wet stuff what's on the ground in the morning?" ("Dew?") "Yeah dew! Well, there's a lot of dew on the grass this morning."

Once children acquire a level of language adequate to function appropriately in their world, they will spend the remainder of their lives using their language to learn more language. Young children have three basic metalinguistic strategies: (1) They use Wh-words in questions; (2) They form hypotheses about how to structure their utterances and test these hypotheses with adult listeners; and (3) They produce utterances that evoke responses from others. We shall discuss each of these strategies.

### Wh-Questions

Children learning to talk often ask lots of questions: "What that?" "Who that?" "Where daddy?" and the all-too-familiar, "Why?" Parents will respond to these questions by supplying the wanted word or explanation, and will probably also correct the question's grammar.

**Child:** "What's that?"

**Parent:** "It's a wheelbarrow. You haul dirt and other things in it. Can you say *'wheelbarrow'*?"

Child:    "bara"

Parent:   "Yes, wheel-barrow"

Child:    "Wee-barrow"

Child:    "Where's daddy?"

Mother:   "Daddy's at work at his office."

Child:    "Daddy at work."

By applying these selective imitation strategies, children learn both new words and new grammatical forms from such interactions.

## Hypothesis Testing

In the early months of learning to produce language, children will often produce an utterance that they are not sure of and add an upward inflection to the end of a word or phrase. Such an inflection makes a word or phrase sound like a question.

Child:    "Daddy office?"

Mother:   "Yes, daddy's at his office. He's working at his job at the office."

Child:    "Daddy working—office"

Child:    "I gots three pennies?"

Father:   "Yes, you've got three pennies—here are two more pennies. Now, you've got five pennies."

Child:    "I've got five pennies."

Father :  "Yes, that right—good!"

Child:    [Looking at picture book with older sister] "Tiger?"

Sister:   "No that's a leopard. A tiger has stripes and a leopard has spots. See? This one is the tiger; and this one is a leopard."

Child:    [Pointing to correct pictures] "That leopard." "There a tiger."

Sister:   "You're right—what a smart boy you are!"

### Evocative Utterances

As you can see from the examples above, children learn much about their language system through the affirmations, corrections, and expansions of their utterances that are built into adult responses to their questions and hypothesis testing. In fact, most children's utterances, even those that may not sound like questions, serve to evoke a response from an older listener. The same types of adult feedback will follow the young child's statement—it is either confirmed or corrected and expanded into mini-tutoring session. In the example above, *tiger* produced with a downward inflection would be just as likely to evoke the same response as "tiger?" with an upward inflection (e.g., "No, that's a leopard; here's the tiger").

Thus, simply by talking a lot, young children ensure that they will have many opportunities to learn about their culture's language system. By talking a lot, children invite feedback and modeling of more correct and more mature language forms that map the child's own meanings. In other words, the more children talk, the more likely they are to develop better language skills. At this stage in child development, silence is *not* golden!

These strategies begin early in the one-word stage of development, and they continue to function effectively throughout the language-learning process. In fact, we still depend on these approaches in adulthood. We never stop trying to learn better and more effective language. We can see that using language to learn more language expands rapidly after the early childhood years. For example, after they learn to read, children learn even more about language from the language used in books. Formal education about the words and rules of syntax that define our language system begins in school. We continue to use words to learn more about our language right through adulthood. We turn to a dictionary or thesaurus to learn about words; and we listen and read to learn more about correct usage of forms, such as *who* vs. *whom*; or *which* vs. *that*.

## THE WORD-LEARNING EXPLOSION

Between 1 year and 2 years of age typical children have learned to play their role in language learning extremely well. They listen, watch, imitate, and try out their language. They also come to know what they can expect from adults—friendly corrections, models for imitation, and expansions of minimal or grammatically inadequate utterances. At this point, they go on a language-learning spree. They can often learn a word with one minimal lesson, and they retain it and use it immediately. This rapid learning of language is helped by the fact that parents are, by now, well attuned to their children's learning style and know exactly what to do to make words and phrases learnable for them.

At this point in the language-learning game, parents begin to search their children's language utterances for more refined teaching targets. For example, they do a lot of test-questioning of their children to see how adequate their vocabulary and grammar are to handle various situations. As they have done from earliest infancy, adults try to respond to children's language efforts positively and constructively. As parents and teachers, we recognize and accept our responsibility to pass on our culture's language system to our children. We know that our children must have an adequate language system if they are to live and succeed among their fellow beings.

## REVIEW AND PREVIEW

In the last three chapters we have looked in some detail at the partnership between the adult teachers and infant learners. We have seen that both parents and children have active and demanding roles in this overall teaching-learning partnership. We have seen, for example, that adults behave in ways that emphasize social interaction and responsiveness to their infant partners. In turn, infants work at participating in these interactions that are modeled by adults. They learn to attend to common foci, respond to turn-taking patterns, and to act on, and respond to, the people, things, and action events in their environment.

Both adults and children have instinctual and learned strategies for optimizing their mutual teaching and learning. We have seen that their respective strategies are complementary. That is, adults behave in ways that facilitate the child's learning of all of the important elements of interaction, physical-world knowledge, and communication. Very young children, then, behave in ways that allow them to use these facilitative adult behaviors to the highest degree possible. In typical families, these behavioral patterns are cooperative, sincere, and constructive among both adults and children. Adults love to see their babies learn and move toward full participation in their social environments. Babies are highly motivated to *program* their powerful brains. They seek sensory and social experiences and they actively process these experiences and create their unique knowledge base. They, basically, actively create their own minds—their private repositories of the carefully constructed knowledge base that is contained in the billions of neuron pathways created in their own particular brain. Of course, this knowledge base reflects the realities of their overall world and, thus, contains much in common with the knowledge of other people in their world. We must realize, however, that no two people have *identical* sets experiences; thus, one person's mind is unique and differs from that of any other person.

Clearly, the overall *quality* of the interactive partnership between children and the caregiving adults in their environment is important to the children's development. Clearly too, the quality of any one child's participation in this partnership affects the final level of his or her learning. This is why both adults and children need to commit totally to these various learning processes. In the next chapter, we will look more carefully at what children are learning during this intense period of language teaching and learning. As you can already imagine, this early learning is basic and sets the stage for a lifetime of future learning. So, let's get to it!

## SUMMARY

- Adults and children have instinctual and learned strategies for optimizing their mutual teaching-learning partnership. Their respective strategies are complementary.

- Infants learn to participate in interactions with adults by attending to common foci, responding to turn-taking patterns, and acting on and responding to the people, things, and action events in their environment.

- Babies must know something about the people, things, or events in their environment before they can learn to comprehend or produce the language by which they can refer to these things. Once they have knowledge of the people, things, and events around them, they must learn to connect the words and phrases they hear to the people, things, and/or events to which the speaker is referring.

- Around 1 year of age, typically developing babies begin to produce language of their own. Through selective listening, they selectively imitate the words that adults emphasize in their talk.

- As children gain increased facility with language, they can use it to form wh-questions, form hypotheses on how to structure their utterances, and produce utterances that evoke responses from their listeners. This enables them to learn language by using language.

- The overall quality of the interactive partnership between children and the caregiving adults in their environment is important to children's development. Similarly, the quality of a child's participation in this partnership affects the final level of his or her learning

## References

Bloom, L. (1970). *Language development: Form and function in emerging grammars.* Cambridge, MA: M.I.T. Press.

Bruner, J. S. (1975). The ontogenesis of speech acts. *Journal of Child Language, 2,* 1–19.

Snyder, L. K., & McLean, J. E. (1977). Deficient acquisition strategies: A proposed conceptual framework for analyzing severe language deficiency. *American Journal of Mental Deficiency, 81,* 338–349.

Snyder-McLean, L., & McLean, J. (1978). Verbal information gathering strategies: The child's use of language to acquire language. *Journal of Speech and Hearing Disorders, 43,* 306–325.

White, R. W. (1959). Motivation reconsidered: The concept of competence. *Psychological Review, 66,* 297–333.

Yarrow, L. J., Morgan, G. A., Jennings, K. D., Harmon, R., & Gaiter, J. L. (1982). Infants' persistence at tasks: Relationships to cognitive functioning and early existence. *Infant Behavior and Development, 5,* 131–141.

# 5

# SUMMARY REVIEW OF CHILDREN'S COGNITIVE LEARNING IN THE PERIOD FROM BIRTH TO 2 YEARS:

# PREPARATION FOR LANGUAGE

## JAMES McLEAN

## Key Concepts

✔ Infants and young children move through specific developmental stages that affect how they respond to their environment and how their environment responds to them.

✔ The cognitive development of infants and young children is best described in terms of the senses and motor movements used to explore and experience their world. Hence, the term sensori-motor development.

---

✔ Cognitive development is linked directly to the use of the senses and motor movement to experience the world, at first reactively and then proactively.

✔ There are four key sensorimotor skills that children use to build their knowledge of people and things that have direct links to language development.

✔ The development of intentional communicative acts is a major precursor to language use.

---

## INTRODUCTION

The etymological roots of the word *cognition* lie in the Latin verb *to know*. In English, the word *cognition* is used to refer to the mental process by which knowledge is acquired, i.e., *learning*. Thus, the term cognitive development is used to refer to both the overall mental process of learning and the products of that process—knowledge.

In previous chapters, we offered details about how adults and children work together in synchronized and complementary ways to begin to teach and learn the knowledge that is crucial to attaining and sustaining a successful life in a complex social and technological environment. In detailing the adult's role in teaching and the child's role of learning, we have already provided the reader with a good look at the kinds of knowledge that children acquire in this intensive process. However, this early knowledge was discussed in rather a piecemeal way. Now it is time to summarize and review, in a more systematic way, the knowledge base that very young babies' acquire from the teaching by the adults and from their own actions on their environment. The reader may feel that much of the following discussion is redundant because much of it has been presented in other contexts in this book. We think, however, that some redundancy functions well to "fix" information in one's knowledge base. And, as we look at linguistic acquisition in the next chapter, we think that having this review of the knowledge that children bring to language learning fresh will be helpful.

So, let's look at some of this again in a more focused way.

# THE NATURE OF EARLY CHILDHOOD COGNITIVE HOLDINGS

The knowledge holdings that are targeted in the earliest teaching and learning processes are those that are rudimentary to all human knowledge. That is, adults first teach and children first learn a limited, but extremely important, body of knowledge about both the people and things of their environment. By mastering a relatively small number of very basic concepts, children are equipped to gather more and deeper levels of knowledge about both their physical and their social worlds. We have talked a bit about some of these early concepts in previous sections of this book. Here, however, we will organize them and provide more details about them so that you can see how basic and profoundly important they are.

We will again apply Bruner's (1975) descriptive categories of "thing skills" and "people skills" to distinguish the two complementary types of knowledge bases that children develop. As you already know, "thing skills" refer to learning that involves elements and attributes of the *physical world*, specifically, infants' learning about the types, attributes, and relationships that exist among physical objects. The term, "people skills" refers to the child's early learning about the social world, the actions, attributes, and relationships that exist among human beings that will allow children to act appropriately on that world. Both of these spheres of knowledge are crucial to the development of a number of specific types of life skills. Furthermore, certain aspects of both the people and thing knowledge tracks *must come together* to enable the acquisition of communication and language. We have noted that children must know a lot about both the people and the physical objects of their environment in order to learn and use language. Thus, although language is the ultimate *people* skill, it cannot be acquired and used until a child has also developed a full repertoire of knowledge about the physical things that make up his or her environment. It is this overall body of knowledge, in both domains, that will be basic to the ability of children to *reference* the elements of their environment by their use of language.

As we apply this two-track organizational framework and discuss these distinct learning domains, we must remember that children are busy acquiring people skills and things skills simultaneously. Thus, there are stages of development for both categories that overlap one another. For this reason, we will discuss what happens to each of these skill categories during each of several stages of development. When we later look at the language that children have developed by the time they are 2½ to 3 years of age, we will be able to see clearly the critical relationship between children's knowledge in both domains.

## THE FIRST 3 MONTHS

During the first 3 months of life, children do not learn concepts as much as they begin to "prime" their millions of brain neurons with experiences and stimuli that can eventually be put together to form concepts. Conceptual learning involves connecting of the information received and stored within and between various neural pathways in different parts of the brain. Thus, before true conceptual learning can be developed, millions of these pathways must be established throughout the brain. These pathways, as we have seen, are established by electrical stimuli sent to the brain from the five senses of vision, hearing, olfactory, touch, and the internal *proprioceptive* stimuli created by one's bodily postures and movements.

### Thing Skills in the Earliest Months of Life

In the period between birth and about 3 months, although babies have five senses, *most* of the stimuli that they experience come to them through the three senses of vision, hearing, and olfactory (taste and smell). Although the senses of touch and proprioception, the internal stimuli that emanate from one's own bodily movements, are intact and also contribute stimuli to babies, these two senses are not as productive as the other senses in these early months because a baby's movements and other motor skills are extremely limited. Very young infants cannot effectively reach, grasp, and release objects. Neither can they coordinate their motor movements to manipulate objects with any degree of purposefulness. They cannot roll over. They cannot locomote. Thus, they cannot create the events that provide particularly rich stimulation to their senses of touch and proprioception. Later in their development, of course, children's active movements and manipulation of objects will create many opportunities for learning. As a result of their early motor limitations, however, a very young baby's energies and efforts are most productively applied in looking at, listening to, and tasting and smelling the environmental objects and events that come into their proximity.

We have seen that parents as well as other adults and children work hard to make up for very young babies' lack of motor skills by bringing much of the world directly to these relatively helpless beings, or by taking them to the sites of action events and sensory experiences. Even with their motor limitations, then, very young babys' brains are being bombarded with impulses from their senses—creating pathways among the neurons that can later be recalled and combined into real knowledge. Research indicates that, at these relatively early stages, children are acquiring notions about familiar versus unfamiliar objects, pleasant sensory stimuli versus unpleasant. We know, too, that even though they lack the good motor control that would allow them to move about and explore their environment, babies are able to use their visual, auditory, and olfactory senses to act on their environment by tracking items and events within it. Very young babies will turn their heads and visually follow an object or person. They will seek out the source of sounds. They very quickly demonstrate preferences for complex patterns of visual and auditory stimuli as opposed to simple patterns. For example, babies very much like to look at human faces. They also like to be talked to, sung to, and cuddled. They like to have objects brought to them so that they can examine them visually. Babies at this stage learn to associate certain scents and odors with certain people, objects, and events. As their senses of touch and taste begin to be stimulated, they seek every opportunity to touch, smell, and taste people and objects. All of these stimuli create pathways in the brain that are used to put together the concepts that will become evident in the ensuing months.

Thus, even when babies are extremely limited in their motor abilities, one look at their eyes, body movements, and facial expressions reveals that they are extremely active in observing and experiencing the world around them. They are clearly learning that there are hundreds of things and events out there in their environment, and they are developing an ability for being able to focus all of their senses on the perception and connecting of those items and events for eventual recall. These small beginnings of collecting stimuli created by the people and things around them allow babies to develop a recognition of recurring items and events and thus create preferences for, and familiarity with, these items or events. This is why that special blanket becomes special and why the Teddy bear becomes a necessity at times of stress. This is why the music box playing, the rattle making noises, and a hanging mobile's actions become such a treat for very young babies. Those of you who have had experience with very young babies know that events such as these will keep babies looking, smiling, kicking, reaching, and making noises.

What babies learn about "things" in the first few months of life is that they provide visual, olfactory, textual (touch), and auditory stimuli, and that these stimuli are interesting. They also begin to be aware that these stimuli can reoccur after they have disappeared for a period of time. Thus, babies have the opportunity to understand what things are more or less permanent elements in their environment. Babies also experience the fact that a moving object can be maintained in their immediate environment, at least for brief periods of time, by a turn of their heads, which allows them to visually or auditorily "track" it. At deeper levels of the human *psyche*, perhaps best labeled as instinct, babies seem to "know" that they must seek out every possible sensory experience. This instinct is powerfully demonstrated by the fact that babies actively seek stimulation from outside themselves and, importantly, that such stimulation seems necessary to keep them happy and active.

## People Skills in the Earliest Months

The lack of the fine motor skills needed for actions on the environment, which inhibits the learning of things skills in the first 3 months, is also a factor in the acquisition of *people* skills at these early stages of development. There are, however, major factors that allow motorically limited infants to experience more intense stimulation from the people element of their environment than the things element. While other people may bring many objects and other physical entities to children to experience, these things are not as compelling to a child's senses as are people themselves. People are simply overwhelming to babies in terms of their stimulus properties. People surround children with stimuli such as touch, warmth, and odors. They bring about gentle pressures on babies' bodies. Their complex facial features with their various expressions provide visual stimuli to babies' brains. People provide movement to babies as they turn them, change them, and carry them about. They provide food. They also bring to babies an almost constant barrage of pleasant-sounding speech. It is no wonder that babies, with their instinctive search for outside stimulation, form quick and lasting affinity to, and preference for, others of their species. What a rich source of experiences the people around them provide.

So what are the most basic "people skills" that very young infants learn and display? First, they learn to be alert to and visually and auditorily attend to people and any actions or objects that people present. They begin to demonstrate the adoption of the common focus with others. They react to other people's efforts to engage them by smiling, cooing, and reaching out to people. They "snuggle." Sometimes, of course, babies will find themselves uncomfortable or unhappy. On these occasions, they may cry loudly until their needs are met; or, if they have had too much stimulation, they may avert their gaze from people and pull away or otherwise resist people's attempts to engage them. They may also stiffen their bodies and squirm, effectively resisting adult comforting caresses.

In summary, in these early months of life, babies form attachments to people and seek out stimulation from them. They reward others for interacting with them both by reacting to events and proactively seeking out visual, touch, and auditory stimulation. They "punish" adults when they are upset by crying or by resisting adult engagement and cuddling. They come to know certain people and demonstrate preferences for them. Their alertness, attention, and reactions provide parallel excitement for the adults around them, thus rewarding caregivers for their efforts. The human instincts for socialization are strengthened by the mutually constructive interplay between adults and babies. Each is stimulated and reinforced by the other as they play out their roles as interactive social beings. It is a wonderful period of connecting and bonding that anticipates the cooperative, giving, and responsive roles that undergird the full socialization to come.

## FOUR TO 9 MONTHS

The next 5 to 6 months of a baby's life are momentous as he or she turns from being primarily a *reactor* to becoming a *proactor*, who is able to motorically act on the objects and people in his or her environment. Although these proactive efforts are necessarily unrefined at the beginning of this developmental period, by its end, babies' motor abilities have developed enough to allow them to truly act on their environment and their learning allows these acts to become purposeful and productive in both the people and thing domains.

### Thing Skills During the Early, Proactive Period

The escalating refinement of young babies' motor skills is absolutely critical to the refinement of their thing skills, because it allows them to create and then *re-create* actions on the objects in their environment. Because thing skills are based on knowledge about the physical elements of the environment and the relationships that obtain between and among these elements, children must experience these things and relationships over and over in order to infer the nature of these entities *and* relationships. When, for example, very young babies flail away at an object displayed on a mobile suspended above their crib and see it move, they do not understand that they caused the movement. Their first instincts are simply to re-create the conditions in which the movement occurred. So, they flail away again. Perhaps this time, however, they do not hit the object attached to the mobile. Not being reinforced for their re-creation of events, a baby might try again or might abandon the activity, not to try again for a day or so. When they are again successful in observing movement of the object, they re-create the flailing activity. As their movements continue to be successful in moving the object they have discovered that they can *re-create* an event that they enjoy and they continue to pursue their new activity. It is not until months later that children discover the fact that their own movements caused the mobile to move about on its string. Think about how profound the notion of cause is as an early concept. First it creates the knowledge about one's ability to "make things happen." Second, it sets up the basis for a child's later awareness about the relationship between *cause* and *effect*. Thus when an event occurs around them in later stages of development, babies look for the *cause* of the event. Early, when they act on a thing, babies look to see, hear, or feel the effects of that act. In the months to follow, this concept of causing things to happen will be a key factor in the acquisition of communicative behaviors, including vocalizations and gestures and, eventually, the final achievement of speech and language.

In another important "thing skill" domain, when very young babies accidentally knock their stuffed animal from their crib, their initial perception is only that it is gone from their environment. However, after experiencing the toy's return, or *recurrence*, many, many times, they begin to get the notion that, even though an item is out of their sight—it still *exists*. This simple discovery is the basis for many, many extremely important learned concepts about the world. For example, the notions that undergird the later development of concepts of "lost," "found," "do it again," and "more" all depend, to some degree, on this awareness that many physical entities continue to exist even when they are out of one's sight or possession. Similarly, babies become aware that, sometimes, an item, such as a certain cookie that they have been eating, is truly "all gone" only until "more" cookies can be coaxed out of mother.

Jean Piaget (1952) identified the basic early childhood concepts that undergird most knowledge about entities in the world and the relationships between and among them. He tracked the gradual development of these basic concepts among typically developing infants and showed how they began with simple discoveries that followed a predictable developmental pattern and culminated in a body of children's early knowledge that he called *sensorimotor skills*. (See Table 5–1 for a listing of Piaget's stages.) We will identify and define several sensorimotor skills a bit later. First, however, let us be aware of and sensitive to the implica-

### Table 5–1
Piaget's Stages of Cognitive Development

| Sensorimotor (0–2 yrs) | Preoperational (2–7 yrs) | Concrete Operational (7–11 yrs) | Formal Operational (11–Adult) |
|---|---|---|---|
| Infants and toddlers: | Preschoolers: | Young students: | Adolescents and adults: |
| Initially rely on reflexive actions. | Initially use words to represent broad categorizations. | Develop ability to consider more than one dimension in problem-solving. | Demonstrate ability to categorize abstract classes and relationships. |
| Repeat interesting actions (primary circular reaction). | Begin categorizing objects through direct paired comparisons. | Reason flexibly by mentally reversing processes. | Demonstrate ability to reason flexibly and verbally through complex problems. |
| Combine existing schemes with new stimuli (secondary circular reactions). | Gradually refine word meanings. | Begin mentally categorizing objects without direct comparisons. | Demonstrate ability to reason through hypothesis testing. |
| Imitate actions they already perform. | Perceive situations from their perspective only (egocentric thought). | | |
| Imitate new actions not previously performed. | Focus on one dimension in problem-solving. | | |
| Demonstrate intention to influence behavior of others (means-end). | | | |
| Actively search for missing objects or persons (object permanence). | | | |
| Play with objects flexibly (symbolic play). | | | |

*Source:* From *Introduction to Language Development*, by S. McLaughlin, 1998, p. 99. San Diego: Singular Publishing Group. Reprinted with permission.

tions of Piaget's label for this body of skills, because he labeled them for the specific abilities that enabled infants to learn these skills—their sensory reception of many types of stimuli and their motor abilities to act on entities in their environment. His key (and profound) point was that young babies are *active* in their learning. Knowledge is not simply "poured into" a child's mind. Rather, it is "discovered" by children from the experiences that they gain through their senses and their actions on entities in their environment. Clearly, Piaget's research findings and perspectives on infants as active in their learning are well demonstrated in the examples of both adult and child actions and strategies in the previous chapter. These perspectives will be prominent in all of the other chapters as well.

### Earliest Schemes for Interacting with Objects

In the first few months of babies' lives, their motor actions on the physical objects they encounter are quite gross. Basically, they tend to carry out a small set of simple action schemes on all objects. They look at them. They mouthe them. They flail at them. If objects are placed in their hands, they will grasp them, shake them, and bang them against the crib, a wall, or their body. They carry out these same actions regardless of the object. This means that a shoe will be mouthed just as readily as a teething ring. Thus, Ina Uzgiris (Uzgiris & Hunt, 1975) has called babies' actions in these early stages *undifferentiated*. In a second stage of this development, however, babies' actions on objects begin to change; they begin to exhibit what Uzgiris called *differentiated actions*. Children begin to do some different things to different objects. Uzgiris observed three behaviors emerging in this stage. The first was an "examining" schema, in which children manipulated an object and examined it visually. The second was the emergence of a preference for acting on objects that were "responsive." Thus, rattles and other noisemakers were manipulated more often than say a stuffed animal. Furthermore, babies seemed to carry out the specific actions that best evoked the responsiveness of an object. Rattles were shaken more than mouthed. Small objects that could be manipulated and thrown or dropped were preferred over large objects that did not allow such acts. The third emerging behavioral schema observed in the later stages of pure infancy was that of coordinating different actions on objects. Thus a ball or block might be examined, banged, mouthed, and then thrown. And late in this coordination of actions stage, babies will begin to use one object on another object, such as banging two blocks together or using a stick to bang on another object. All of these developmental attainments culminate in action schemas that are highly differential among different objects. Thus, as babies learn that certain objects respond more to some types of actions than to others, they begin to narrow their action schemes on certain objects to those to which the object best responds.

### Advanced Schemes for Objects

Young children have acquired a rich repertoire of differentiated actions on objects by around 9 months of age. They are now ready to try to "master" the physical things in their world. Thus, they set out to refine their actions on objects according to two primary guidelines. First is the aforementioned "affordance" properties of the objects they encounter (i.e., what does one do with a certain object to create the most interesting or productive response from that object?). Do you shake it, bang it, throw it, stack it, nest it in another object, roll it, or taste it? Do you push it, pull it, or drop it on the floor? Do you listen to its noise, feel its texture, or just look at it? Babies, through their own experimentations, then, learn what actions on various objects best afford in terms of how the objects react to various types of actions on them. They then tend to carry out the *differential action schemes* that best fit the object. They begin to use these specific schemes consistently with familiar favorite objects. Thus, balls begin to be rolled or thrown; blocks begin to be stacked on one another; and mobiles above the crib begin to be hit with tiny hands and watched carefully.

### Coordinated Actions on Objects

Once babies begin to learn what actions work best on certain objects, they often find themselves with two objects at hand, and the new challenge becomes how to use these two objects together. Can they be made to act on one another to some good result? Probably the first coordinated action with two objects is to bang them together. Certainly this produces interesting effects if done with two blocks—or a stick and a *Tinker Toy* box. Certainly the fun of putting small blocks or other toys into some box or bottle is an interesting new scheme, as is the action of shaking the box after the blocks or Legos have been placed inside, and later pouring the contents out of the bottle or box.

By 9 to 12 months, typically developing children have learned to sit up, crawl, and often walk. As a result of these new skills, they have become quite active in their play with things in their environment. They have learned to get a real "bang from their buck," as it were. They can make things happen and then make them happen again at will. At this stage children are grasping and manipulating objects with some degree of skill, although they still lack truly "refined" fine motor skills. We will look at what happens in the next 9 months a bit later. For now, however, we want to look at the parallel development of "people skills" in this stage between 3 months and 9 months of age.

## People Skills Learned During the Early Proactive Period

During this period where children's improving motor skills allow them to be able to act on objects in their environment, we see concomitant progress in their abilities to act on people as well. With their vision improving and their strong instincts to focus on people, babies now maintain almost constant visual contact with people who are in their immediate environment. They look for opportunities to engage other people in some interaction. In the early months of this stage, these engagements might only be establishing joint focus with the adult and, perhaps, an object that the adult has or is attending to. The adult most often talks to the baby and acts on him or her, or on the object in some way, and then pauses. Babies at this stage have developed some rudimentary feel for the give-and-take pattern of human interactions, so they begin to "fill their turn" in the interaction, usually by making a sound or acting physically with a reach or smile. Or perhaps the baby simply begins to kick to indicate that he or she is into the interaction. When the adult then takes his or her turn, the standard reciprocal pattern of interactions is maintained for as long as the baby and the adult are willing to play. At this stage too, babies will usually attempt to reach and grasp any object that the adult brings to the interaction.

In the later months of this stage (around 7 months), typically developing children will be able to sit up and can visually guide their reach to touch adults and toys alike. This is the stage when children begin to touch adults' faces, tug at their glasses and hair, and both give and take objects from their play partner. At this point the turn-taking responses are emerging strongly and adults feel that their child is truly becoming a partner in their interactions. Children listen to adult speech and begin to comprehend frequently heard speech signals for games such as peek-a-boo and other simple reciprocal, give-and-take games. Babies' smiles and noises of glee, excitement, or unhappiness are frequent in this stage. It is in this stage too, that babies begin to react to other speech signals like "no" and "stop," particularly when they are uttered louder and sharper than the adult's usual tone.

Although we will discuss it in more detail later in this chapter, we might note here that it is in this stage that adults begin to "read" children's actions and noises and begin in earnest to "assign" communicative significance to them. Thus, when a baby hands an object to an adult, the adult makes a judgment about why the baby has done so. Does the baby want a music box wound up or does he or she want a demonstration about how to act on this particular item? The adult then acts in accordance with his or her decision about what the baby "intended" by his or her actions. If they have guessed wrong, and the baby repeats the action or acts frustrated, adults will usually recalculate their guess as to the baby's intent and act in accordance with another assumption.

By the time a child reaches 9 months of age or so, he or she is close to being a true, proactive, turn-taking, and responsive interactive partner. While the months ahead will produce more and better social interaction skills, including intentional communication and language, the typical 9-month level of development reveals the social nature of very young children and their clear appreciation for the adult's presence and role in their lives. A personality has emerged in babies; and their adult caregivers and play partners can see that they are poised to enter fully into social living. It is a fun time for all.

## NINE TO 18 MONTHS: (THE TODDLER STAGE)

In the vernacular, it is in these next 9 months that children really begin to "make hay" in both the thing and people domains. In the toddler stage, typically developing children become dramatically more skilled in their motor abilities and are able to act more purposefully on the physical world. They learn to crawl and then

walk and, with these new abilities, can move to purposefully access things in the world. They also have hours upon hours to manipulate and examine objects. They can experiment with various
actions on them. They can feel them, throw them, roll them, taste
them, and listen to the noises they might make. Now, they can
combine them to make new entities. They stack things, put one
thing in another, hide things, and then retrieve them.

## The Most Basic Sensorimotor Skills Learned in the Toddler Stage

The behavioral repertoires for acting on the world that young
children display during the period between 9 and 18 months are
*not* just rote imitations of the actions they have observed other
people perform. To be sure, children have learned some actions
on objects by observing others. Often, however, they don't truly
understand the reason for these actions. For example, toddlers
will often put a string of beads around their necks. This act has
no function to the child except as it reflects something that Mommy does. Similarly, the awful job of putting on shoes and socks
seems to have no purpose other than "it is something that is
done." Other items of clothing also seem to be seen as "optional"
to most babies, who are just as happy to be unencumbered by
clothing. It is only much later that children understand social
conventions such as modesty and protection from the elements
that set up the need for clothing. The functions of such things as
beads, earrings, and makeup as attempts to enhance personal
style or beauty are not clearly understood by young children. Yet
such actions are often found in their behaviors because they seem
to be important to the adults around them.

The latter concepts are purely social and, in a way, might be
classed as people skills that are carried out with objects. However, during this period, babies learn many other nonsocial schemes
for objects during this period that reflect truly important concepts about the physical world and their place in it, concepts that
will allow them to understand and use the entities of their physical world to both sustain and better their lives. Jean Piaget (1952)
categorized *six* key concepts in this sensorimotor domain. In the
following discussion, we will be emphasizing *four* of them. The
four that we will discuss in detail were chosen because they ap-

pear to relate most specifically to language *form, content,* and *use* and the knowledge bases needed for each of these elements. When we look specifically at the language that emerges in the toddler stage, the importance of these four sensorimotor concepts will be readily apparent.

### Object Permanence

We have all experienced the frustration of a very young infant when a favorite toy is inadvertently covered up by a blanket in the crib. The young infant doesn't search for the object—rather he or she simply assumes the object is "gone" and either forgets it or cries in frustration at its disappearance. An infant's discovery that an object or person that has been removed from his or her immediate perception still exists in the physical world is a crucial one. We have already noted that this concept of object permanence undergirds the meanings carried in many early words such as "allgone," "more," and "again." It is also the keystone for many other concepts that are important for intelligent living in the physical world. It allows a baby to search for a lost toy and to develop preferences for favorite objects and toys that he knows can be readily accessed. It fosters forethought in solving problems, because it allows babies to conceptualize an object needed in a particular situation and to retrieve it (e.g., Is a cup needed for the tea party? Fine, I'll get one from the toy chest and while I'm there I'll also get the spoons. Is "Fluffy" missing? That's okay— "Fluffy" still exists and can be reaccessed in the future. Maybe he's in my bed).

These examples show how this very basic concept of object permanence provides the bases for other quite basic concepts such as "existence," "nonexistence," "location," and "possession." As such, then, this single concept provides the knowledge bases for certain actions and action plans, as well as the meanings and need for many, many future words. Later in this book, when we look specifically at the early words that most children learn and use first, we will see that many of them are related to the concepts as emanating from the notion of object permanence.

### Means to Desired Ends

As children operate on various elements of their environment during this highly active period, they begin to discover the relationships between their own behaviors and the behaviors of the objects in this environment. In their early months, babies might recognize that there is a relationship between one of their actions and an object event. However, their full understanding of this relationship is not yet developed. To very young babies, most events are rather magical. As they refine their actions on objects to those that bring them the most response from the objects, however, they begin to discover that they can behave in ways that make *predictable things* happen with those objects. The more experience they have in carrying out operations on objects, the more creative and successful they become in attaining results that they desire. They begin by knocking down towers of blocks their daddy builds and then stack their own towers to demolish. They learn to use a stick to retrieve a toy that is out of their reach. They learn to wind things up and to turn on the various switches that their toys require to perform actions or produce noise. They learn to remove or go around objects that block their movements.

By 18 months of age most children are able to operate on their physical environment with an amazing number of strategies and behaviors. They can use rudimentary toy tools and they can *preplan* a course of action. They have developed a sense of what to do to obtain a desired result from the things in their physical environment. When we look at communication and language development in the next chapter, we will see that this ability to design certain means to attain desired ends in the physical world is matched by the concomitant development of the socio-communicative behaviors by which desired ends can be best attained from other people. Indeed, babies must be able to make things happen with all of the entities that inhabit their world, and they are working like mad to learn all of the ways to do so.

### Causality

This busy, busy period of making things happen finally brings babies to the point where they understand the notion of consequences that stem from their actions. They come to understand that these consequences are predictable and, thus, can be repeated with rather consistent results. This discovery is the basic element in understanding causes and effects among entities in their environment. Thus, when children experience an "effect," they look for the "cause." Even more so, they now can consider an effect that they desire to occur and develop a plan about how to cause that effect.

This discovery certainly emanates from their development of "schemes for objects" and "means to desired ends" but clearly goes beyond them. The notion of causality is now a concept that allows children to intelligently plan behavioral schemes to obtain ends that they desire. A full understanding of the notion of cause and effect results in an ability to conceptualize a desired end and, then, to conceptualize a plan of action to obtain that end. Children will use a stick to pull a small toy out of a cage; and they will throw other toys out of their way to retrieve a desired toy that is at the bottom of their toy basket. They have come a long way from their early attempts to bat at a mobile over the crib, knocking down block towers, and even knowing that a telephone is placed up to one's ear. Toddlers have gained the power to seek out objects and events that *they* desire. That is why the "terrible two's" are so terrible. Babies have become enamored by their newly discovered power to make things happen in both their physical and social worlds—and they begin to use it with both gusto and persistence!

This constellation of *object schemes*, besides serving children in their immediate activities, also sets up opportunities to better understand events in the environment that they observe. Thus, this concept undergirds a child's understanding of the different types of actions one can take to make an event happen. They learn that you can *push, pull, pry, twist,* or *turn* an object. They watch mother in the kitchen and begin to understand the basic notions of cooking a meal or ironing clothes. In the most basic sense, young children discover the action worlds of work, creative activities, and play. Thus they begin to acquire the knowledge-directed behavioral repertoires that allow them to function effectively and productively in all of the different contexts of the physical environment that they encounter. This learning enables children to further develop their repertoire of specific skills. Even further, it sets up their motivation to continue to learn the additional skills that will be needed to solve future problems. It alerts them to the fact that every situation requires them to have special skills in order to function effectively and productively. Thus, it sets them on the track for seeking further knowledge and skills throughout their lives. Because of their successes in the development of the basic sensorimotor skills, children are confident and motivated to continue their efforts to master the world around them.

## Conventional Schemes on Objects and the Emergence of Symbolic Play

After all of this experience with things in their environment, children have greatly narrowed the sets of actions that they apply to certain things. They waste little time in choosing to apply only the most productive action schemes to their toys. In addition to conducting their personal experimentation on objects, young babies also observe other people's actions on objects. Because many objects or entities exist to perform some useful function, babies must depend on other people to show them what these various functions are. At this stage, babies are ready to begin imitating the actions they see adults and other children carry out. Thus, they hammer with hammers, roll balls and cars, and turn pages in books. It is in this stage that children will begin to "pretend" to drink from an empty cup, put mother's shoes on their feet, and put her strings of her beads around their neck. They will also begin to feed their dolls from toy nursing bottles, hold a phone to their ear and vocalize, and pretend to be eating imaginary cookies that mother has "given" them. They begin to "stir" in pans rather than bang them. As you can see from these examples, babies are now able to imbue *symbolic representations* of real items (i.e., models, pictures, and word-names) with all of the attributes of the *actual item*. Thus, as they push toy trucks and cars, they will make vocal noises that represent the sounds of their engines and they will make them stop , go, back up, and screech to a stop. When they hear a word such as "baby," they will get their doll and proceed to hug it, rock it, or comb its hair.

This pretend play is called "symbolic play" and it is a major milestone in a baby's development for several reasons. First, symbolic play reveals that a baby now understands that an item or action can be "represented" by some item or action that is not, strictly speaking, the item or action itself. Babies know that a doll is not a real baby and that the toy, miniature bottle from which they feed the doll is not a real bottle of milk. They also know that their pretend tea party is only a representation of the real thing. This ability to let something that is *not* the real thing *represent* the real thing is a crucial discovery for children. It is this unique abili-

ty that allows pictures and drawings to be useful, lets pantomimic gestures be understood, and undergirds and makes possible
the eventual use of language to *represent* items, actions, and events
of the real world. Indeed this ability to create and understand
symbolic representations is the one of the most crucial hallmarks
of human intelligence. It is the unique ability that makes all of
our advanced systems of oral and written languages and mathe-
matics possible. It allows the human animal to refer to people,
physical entities, and events that are not in his or her immediate
environment and, thus, allows people to make references to past
and future events.

With the ability to imitate and play symbolically, children
are now able to begin to develop a repertoire of behaviors that reflect and *represent* the events they see in the environment around
them. When we realize that most children also begin to walk and
talk during this period between 9 and 18 months, we can understand parents' feelings that their baby is now becoming a "person." Their baby can now begin to do many of the things that
others in the environment do and, thus, begins to occupy a real
place in the everday world of the people around him or her.
Their baby is becoming both competent in dealing with the physical world and a highly socialized being. It is a great stage in a
child's development for both adults and the child.

As toddlers gain the skills needed to operate successfully on
the world of physical things and other people, they become more
and more aware of their *need* for the other people in their environment. Because they need people to provide models of needed
skills, to encourage and reward them, and to set up the environment so that they can learn and practice these skills, children become increasingly aware of their need to develop their skills for
dealing effectively and productively with those other people.
Thus, in parallel with their developing thing skills, toddlers also
seek to learn and refine their people skills. Indeed they make
great strides in developing their people skills in the toddler stage.
We shall look at these gains in the sections that follow.

## People Skills Emerging in the Toddler Stage

By the time they reach 18 months of age, typically developing
children have the rudiments of social interaction with other peo-

ple well in hand. Obviously, then, between the ages of 9 to 18 months, they have much to learn about how to interact more effectively and efficiently. By 18 months, toddlers who are developing typically will have acquired the rudiments of language. However, there are some important nonlanguage, people skills to learn in the developmental stages prior to that important milestone. Several of these nonlanguage skills are, however, directly related to their future development of language. Foremost among these skills are those that relate to the discovery, understanding, and refinement of the notion of *communication* itself.

At the beginning of the toddler stage (9–10 months of age) we know that children do have a good start in development of people skills. Indeed, they interact regularly and relatively effectively with adults. They pay attention to adults, establish a common focus with them, and are beginning to wait and take turns in interactions. They laugh, initiate games, and demonstrate anger and frustration. At this point in their development, children are quite skilled at making things happen in their physical world. They can also have effects on people through their use of direct actions such as pulls and tugs on them. Their attention to and their direct actions on objects also evoke reactions and constructive responses from other people. However, we must not forget that, despite their significant skills for *directly* acting on things and people, at the beginning of this developmental period, babies are still dependent on attentive careproviders to attend to their actions and *assign* potential communicative significance to them. Having assigned such communicative significance to a baby's acts on them or on some object, interactive partners can then react in the way they deem most appropriate. If they have correctly inferred the intentions of a baby's actions, things are fine and the baby is "satisfied" with their response. If, however, their interpretation of the intentions signaled by the baby's actions is *not* correct, their response does not satisfy the baby and further negotiations are needed. This basic guesswork process can become frustrating for both adults and children. Fortunately, the awarenesses that babies are gradually developing during their interactions with people lead the way to one more stage of people skill development before true language begins to emerge. This last stage involves the baby's development of a set of prelinguistic communicative signals that babies *direct to adults with the intention of evoking certain responses from them.*

## The Development of Intentional Communicative Acts Before Language

We are aware that by 9 months typically developing babies are socialized in that they seek out others to interact with. Babies are also working diligently to acquire more knowledge about their environment. This means that they look more and more for adult or sibling help in acquiring this knowledge. They come to realize that they must have access to more demonstrations and instructions from the people around them who have the skills that they lack. This need fuels their drive to become more and more effective in evoking all sorts of interactions from others. Babies find that they simply must develop more effective and efficient behaviors for evoking desired responses from others. Because the rudimentary behaviors for attaining these needed ends are already present in their repertoires, it remains only for the adult-child partnership to refine them. There are three major steps in this refinement process:

1. Children learn to use *objects* to evoke actions from others;
2. Children learn to issue nonlanguage communicative signals *intentionally*; and,
3. Children learn to utilize *communicative gestures*.

### Use of Objects On People

In babies' earliest interactions with adults and older siblings, we know that the giving and exchanging of objects play an important role in turn-taking routines. From the earliest days of infancy, adult caregivers have been bringing objects into children's view and making them available for them to grasp, mouthe, and otherwise manipulate. In turn, when children have mastered the motor skills necessary to allow them to grasp and then release objects, children begin to reciprocate these exchanges. At first, the giving of an object to an adult is simply an element in their turn-taking ritual. Soon, however, children discover that the giving of an object to an adult usually results in some action by the adult. For example, when given a rattle, the adult might shake it and produce its distinctive noise. Later, adults will respond to an object given to them by demonstrating to the child how the object should be used in terms of either its *affordance* properties or its real-world use. Babies quickly discover that giving an object to an adult routinely results in any of several actions by the adult. As indicated in the examples above, these actions include demonstrations of an object's potential for producing auditory or visual events, its tactile properties (softness, vibratory sensations), and, as noted above, its potential for producing actions that can be seen, heard, or both. Babies rather quickly discover that the adults' demonstrations of an object's physical properties, potential for producing actions, and its real world uses are, in a word, *predictable*. When babies recognize this predictability, they gain increased awareness of an adult's usefulness in proving all sorts of *information* and *problem-solving* help. Thus begins the emergence of a child's deliberate use of objects *on* adults to evoke these acts from them. The deliberate use of objects to evoke actions from adults, then, serves as an act that a child can use for all sorts of purposes as he or she sets out to master the physical world. The use of objects on adults brings a baby an adult's attention, interaction, and, most of all, a wide variety of learning opportunities and pleasures.

In the mind of the adult, these acts with objects by their baby create an awareness of the child as a real, reciprocal partner. Remember, up to now, most of the *proactive* behaviors have been the responsibility of the adult. Babies have simply been the receivers of adults' intense efforts to foster interactions with them. When babies become proactive themselves and use objects on adults, caregivers finally recognize that their relationship with their baby has changed dramatically and productively into a partnership for work, play, and further learning. A truly major *people skill* has been acquired.

### Discovery of Intentional Communication

With their newly discovered awareness that they can use objects to evoke actions from others, children now possess some very profound knowledge, namely, that *people can be acted on just as objects can*. Furthermore, *people will respond to actions on them* just as objects do. A tug on daddy's arm will bring his attention to the tugger. Taking mommy's hand and placing it on a music box will have the same effect that handing her the music box has—Mommy will somehow act on the music box. She will probably wind it up and make it perform its action of producing those pleasant noises. As these skills for having effects on their partners are refined, babies discover that, often, it takes only a look in the direction of a music box or some other toy to evoke some helpful action from their partners.

As the full realization of this new skill comes to a baby, he or she is rather quick to expand it and *use it*. The child now understands that he or she can have a need and can *intentionally* act on a partner to satisfy that need. After all of the months in which parents and other caregivers had to observe a baby's actions and states and *interpret* and *assign* their potential communicative value, partners can now reliably expect a *direct* indication of a child's desire and communicative intentions. Conversely, the baby has found an *efficient* and *effective* way of evoking actions from partners. Babies can now *act* on their partners and *wait* for the usually predictable result of their actions.

This *coordination* of two people's attentions and actions is the most basic use of language in human societies. This is the very function of language that has enabled the development of entire human societies—and it starts with a very young baby and a responsive adult communicative partner! It starts even before language is learned. What a momentous event for both children and their caregivers—*intentional communicative acts* have been discovered.

To be sure, intentional communication can still be ambiguous and, thus, are not always successful. But both caregivers and babies work on making it more effective. As in the past, adult partners first try to understand the *intentions* of a child's act on them. They do this by following a child's line of regard. Do his or her eyes signal the object of the communicative act? Does he use an object on his parent? Next they review the context of their interaction—the here and now of the activity. Is something missing? Is something not working? Is information needed by the child? The adult partner makes his or her choice of possible child intentions and makes a response, watching for the child's reaction. If the choice is correct, the child responds positively and accepts the partner's actions. If the partner has guessed wrong, the child has a number of ways to signal that fact. First, he or she can repeat the previous communicative act. For example, look again at the music box that is not playing, touch it, and look again at the partner. If the adult still does not respond in the way that the child desired, he or she might *back up* to a previously learned communicative skill and hand the music box to the partner. Finally, the partner correctly infers the child's intentions, and responds appropriately. Clearly, there is a lot more learning to be accomplished before communication is truly efficient, so the next phase of communication skill learning begins. And, it is *still not language* that is acquired. Rather, toddlers nearing a year of age begin to refine their actions on both people and objects to develop a set of *gestures* that make their communicative messages more easily understood by their communicative partners.

## The Development of Communicative Gestures

In addition to talking to their young babies, parents have also been making body, hand, and head gestures to their babies from the very beginning of their interactions. These gestures accompany adult talk to children and have been used, for example:

1. When *requesting* objects (extend open hand toward child with the palm up)

2. When *directing the child's attention* to things or events by pointing to things or showing them objects (holding and extending an object in front of the child but *not* giving it to them)

3. When *giving* objects to the child (holding up an object and extending it and letting the child grasp and take it)

4. When waving "bye-bye" or motioning for a child to "come here"

5. When nodding "yes" or "no"

Caregivers use these gestures to augment or supplement their spoken language to increase the probability that the child can learn to comprehend what the words they are hearing mean.

As children are learning to comprehend the *words* being spoken to them, they are also learning to comprehend the *gestures* being used. Children are more and more able to read the "tone" of the adult's language. They discriminate between nice singsongy utterances and more imperative-sounding directions and requests. Certainly, they discriminate angry speech. In fact, children are beginning to reflect their emotions in some of their own nonlinguistic vocalizations. As children's *comprehension* of the various nonlinguistic communicative aspects of adult behavior increases, they begin to develop their own repertoires of such behaviors.

Learning to produce different gestures begins rather soon after comprehension develops. Children of 8 to 10 months can already do the things with their hands and fingers that early gestures require. They can already hold objects, drop objects, extend objects, and reach for things with their fingers extended. The first step in the movement to specific communicative gestures, then, typically involves gestures that are made with an *object in hand*. For example, the grasp becomes a communicative *give gesture* when an object is extended toward another person and is released to that person. The same grasp becomes a *show* gesture when the child extends an object—but declines to let go of it. It is important to note that, when these gestures with objects begin to occur, the child indicates some expectation that the adult will *do* something in response to the gesture. They do this by maintaining eye contact with the receiver, vocalizing, and *waiting*—as adult behaviors for all of these months have taught them to do. If no response is forthcoming from the receiver, the child may repeat the gesture or produce a more emphatic vocal sound. The child might also touch the adult's hand or offer an exaggerated shift of his or her gaze between the adult and the object that is the joint focus in their interaction.

These first gestures with objects are generally used by children to *request* some object or desired adult action on an object. For example, when a child's music box runs down, he or she may *give* the box to an adult to rewind. If a child cannot open a can of blocks, he or she might hand it to an adult or another child to perform the act. This is, basically, a *give for help* gesture. This is often the first gesture a child uses. Other gestures, however, come rapidly. Some gestural acts are carried out directly on others. A child will *tug* on mother's skirt to request attention or take her hand and put it on an object with which he or she needs help. Often children will provide a little gestural demonstration (pantomime) of what should be done with the object (e.g., "open it," "wind it"). Obviously, in most cases, receivers are only happy to oblige the child's requests. They demonstrate an object's function, they open, they rewind, they put parts of a toy together—

delighted to help the child learn about the things at hand. In these situations, adults are again showing children that they are attentive and ready to respond to their communicative efforts.

### Emergence of Distal Gestures

You will note that these earliest child gestures involve making direct contact with an object or person. As such, these first gestures are simply extensions and refinements of the direct motor acts that children previously developed to act on objects and people. They grasp and hold out an object. They tug at mother's hand or skirt. They take a receiver's hand and put it in place on a wind-up toy that isn't performing correctly. We (McLean, McLean, Brady, & Etter, 1991) have called these *contact* gestures because they involve direct child contact with objects and people Later in the gestural stage, children gain the ability to produce the same hand movements but *without an object*. Gestures of this type are called *distal gestures* because they are distanced from referent objects. For example, children begin to produce an open-hand *reach* for things that are some distance from them. As gestural development proceeds, this open-handed reach action is modified in two ways to become two different gestures. At first, children's reaching movements involve the hand being extended with all fingers extended. In the earliest stages of gesture development this open-handed reach (often with fingers wiggling) is often used both as a *request* and a *point*. Later this reaching movement is modified into an open-palm reach with for *requesting* and a closed hand with one finger extended for *pointing*. A refined, "true" point, along with "pantomimic" and "acting out" gestures such as those twisting gestures that we understand to request that we "open this bottle" or "wind this up" finally emerge. These major steps in the young child's development of prelinguistic communication are summarized in Table 5–2.

At this point, children are full-fledged social, communicative beings. Although their nonlanguage communicative repertoire is limited and often inefficient, it is usually effective in bringing about the responses children desire from others. Clearly, however, both children and their caregiving partners are aware that communication between them must become both more effective and more precise. Both adults and children are ready to mount the major push into the acquisition of spoken language.

## Table 5–2

The Evolution of Child Behaviors that Have Communicative Effects on Others

| Order of Emergence and Name | Description of Behaviors | Effects on Other People |
|---|---|---|
| 1. *Reactive actions* | Sucking on hand; rubbing eyes; yawning; "fussing"; stretching | Observers *assign meaning*: "You're hungry; You're sleepy; Are you wet? Oh my, that stretch feels good doesn't it?" |
| 2. *Proactive actions on people or objects* | Reaches for object; touches other person's face; shakes rattle; drops block | Again, observers *assign meaning*: "Do you want that Teddy bear? Aaah, you love daddy don't you? Oops, block all gone—shall I get it? More block?" |
| 3. *Contact gestures:* Direct physical contact made with object or person and action is directed toward another person and a response is expected. | Holds out object to person and allows object to be taken *(Give)*; Extends object to person and *does not* allow it to be taken *(Show)*; Takes person's hand and places it on toy *(Request help or comment)*; Reaches and touches object *(Request object)* | *Child has intentions to communicate (have effects on others) so partner responds in accordance with his or her best understanding of child's intentions.* "Oh, thank—you. I love this Teddy bear. Yes, I see your rattle—can you make it rattle? Ah yes, you want me to wind your music box don't you? Okay, I'll wind it up. Let's let it play now." |
| 4. *Distal gestures:* No direct contact made with object or person. Gesture is "distanced" from referent. | Reaches toward object with fingers outstretched *(Requests attention to object or requests object)*; Holds out hands to person *(Requests action from person,* e.g., pick me up); Waves "bye-bye"; Holds out empty hands and looks at person ("All gone" or "Where is the toy I had?") Points at object *(Direct attention)* | *Child intends to communicate—partner responds in accordance with his or her best understanding of child's intentions.* "You like that music box don't you? Okay, let's make it play. Do you want to hold it up to your ear? Bye-bye baby. Mamma's going bye-bye; Where is it? Is it 'allgone'? Let's find it okay? Here it is. Yes, I see the airplane." |

**Table 5–2** (continued)

| Order of Emergence and Name | Description of Behaviors | Effects on Other People |
|---|---|---|
| 5. *Both contact and distal gestures* supplemented with vocalizations that are "intonated" but not yet recognizable as real words | Reaches toward object and grunts; Hands music box to partner and "fusses"; Hands doll to partner; Hands toy to partner; Extends open palm toward partner | *Child intends to communicate such things as:*<br>• give me/look at that<br>• wind it up<br>• play dolly<br>• fix that<br>• give me |
| 6. *True point and pantomimic gestures* | Points with one finger extended—does not touch referent. This is the final gesture to emerge and is often accompanied by other pantomimic gestures and vocalizations. Pantomimic gestures include: "Take off; put on; wind up; unscrew lid," etc. | *Child intends to communicate* —the point gesture is often accompanied by other gestures, pantomimes, and vocalizations to communicate meanings such as those above and many others. |

# REVIEW AND PREVIEW

As we have seen, the development of nonlinguistic child communicative behaviors begins with two levels of children's actions, *reactive* and *proactive*, to which caregivers *assign* communicative intentions. This assignment or inference of communicative significance to a child's states and, later, actions occurs before a child understands his or her abilities to communicate. This consistent assignment of communicative significance, and adult's responses to such inferences, helps babies to *discover* their ability to have effects on others. Thus, they begin to use actions directly on partners and on objects. These purposeful actions make it easier for partners to interpret a child's needs and to respond to them. The developmental process continues with the emergence and refinement of intentional communicative gestures, which are derived from motor acts that children have previously applied to objects and to people (i.e., *contact* gestures). Children refine these gestures to the point that they can be produced without making direct contact with objects or people, thus, *distal* gestures are developed.

As we consider this period in a child's life and the skills and knowledge that they must gain to go much beyond this stage of development, we quickly realize that children cannot or will not be able to go much farther in their learning or social development until they learn to use *spoken language*. They need language to learn more about their complex physical world and they need language to learn and behave more productively and appropriately in their social world of other people. It is the ability to understand and produce oral language that will allow them to acquire more complex knowledge—knowledge that goes beyond the here and now experiences that they have been able to communicate about up to this point in their life.

The important thing is that both children and parents come to realize the fact that, at some point, language is now necessary, and both make new commitments to teach and learn it. Children bring the same proactive, focused, and energetic efforts to the job of learning language that they previously applied to learning about their physical world of things and people. Adults bring the same efforts to facilitating children's learning of language that they brought to all of the earlier interactions where they facilitated their children's development of nonlanguage knowledge.

Throughout this book, we have talked about various examples of young children's learning , but we have not presented detailed examples of the language-learning process itself. In the next chapter, we will discuss the specifics of a child's language development. As you will see, the process is logical and easy to understand now that we have looked at the kinds of life experiences and learning that children have acquired before they actually come to language. The reader can probably anticipate how some of the learning that precedes language is reflected in the linguistic forms that children learn and the things that they do with it. Hopefully, this review has contributed to an even deeper appreciation of the fact that a baby's linguistic learning is deeply rooted in his or her knowledge holdings prior to learning the language itself. knowledge-holdings that are broad, basic, and necessary for mastering an environment that is both social and physical and knowledge that has required the best cooperative efforts of both adults to teach and children to learn. That knowledge now enables them to acquire and use the most elegant and effective people skill—spoken language.

## SUMMARY

- The development of nonlinguistic communicative behaviors begins with two levels of children's actions, reactive and proactive, to which caregivers assign communicative intention.

- Consistent assignment of communicative significance and adults' responses to such inferences helps babies discover their ability to have effects on others by using actions directly on partners and objects.

- The developmental process continues with the emergence and refinement of intentional communicative gestures, which are derived from motor acts that children have previously applied to objects and people.

- The cognitive development that takes place between birth and 2 years of age is facilitated by children's interactions with adults and with the world around them, but to move beyond this stage of development, children need to learn spoken language.

- What children learn and how they have learned about their physical world of things and people will have a direct influence on the first linguistic forms that children produce.

## References

Bruner, J. S. (1975). The ontogenesis of speech acts. *Journal of Child Language, 2,* 1–19.

McLean, J. E., McLean, L. K. S., Brady, N. C., & Etter, R. (1991). Communication profiles of two types of gesture using nonverbal persons with severe to profound mental retardation. *Journal of Speech and Hearing Research, 34,* 294–308.

Piaget, J. (1952). *The origins of intelligence in children.* New York: W. W. Norton.

Uzgiris, I., & Hunt, J. M. (1975). *Assessment in infancy.* Urbana: University of Illinois Press.

# CHILDREN'S
# EARLY LINGUISTIC
# LEARNING

## JAMES McLEAN

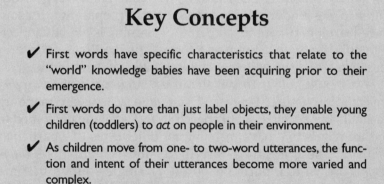

## Key Concepts

✔ First words have specific characteristics that relate to the "world" knowledge babies have been acquiring prior to their emergence.

✔ First words do more than just label objects, they enable young children (toddlers) to *act* on people in their environment.

✔ As children move from one- to two-word utterances, the function and intent of their utterances become more varied and complex.

✔ The two- and three-word stage of language development marks the emergence of grammar.

✔ Language development beyond the three-word utterance stage is characterized by continued vocabulary growth and the refinement of syntactical skills, conversation skills, and speech sound development.

## INTRODUCTION

Since the beginning of this book we have stressed that one cannot fully understand the language development of young children without understanding all of the teaching and learning that goes on *before* language is acquired. In the preceding five chapters we have discussed this preparation for language learning in some detail and from several perspectives. We looked at the roles of parents and other adults and older children in the *socialization* and *cognitive* development of the young child. We detailed the behaviors of the people in the child's environment who already know language as they help children to learn to *comprehend* language. We also looked at how these people specifically aid children in their acquisition of the *linguistic* forms used in their native language. We discussed the strategies of young infants as they work to learn all that is being taught to them. And we reviewed the social patterns and cognitive holdings that children acquire in all of this intensive interaction with the people and physical entities in their environment. Now we are about to examine the linguistic forms that young children learn first. As we look at this early linguistic learning, we think that it will be much clearer to the reader why we stressed this preparation for language-learning. All of this preparatory learning is directly reflected in children's new linguistic forms, the *meanings* carried in these forms, and the uses that children make of these forms.

We should note here that all human language systems are *recombinative* in nature. That is, all language systems are made up of a small, but specific, set of speech sounds that are combined to produce words that have meaning for other users of a particular language. These meaning-carrying sound combinations (*morphemes*) are words, parts of words, or single sounds that are themselves combined to produce other meanings. For example, an /s/ or /z/ is combined with many words to signal that the word is *plural*. The word-part *non* is added to precede such words as *partisan, sense,* and *caring* to signal that the state represented by the word is negated. Even further, then, these words are combined in phrases and sentences that can be used to express all kinds of meaningful communicative acts.

All of these meaningful units of sounds are then used to have effects on other people. As we have discussed, language is used to conduct the complex social business of humans; the business that allows them to live cooperatively and productively among others of their species.

Thus, in this chapter, as we look at the early language development of young children, we will see each of the components of a complex, three-level linguistic structural system emerge and be used as a social tool.

## THE BEGINNINGS OF
## LINGUISTIC FORMS AND THEIR USE

By 1 year of age, typically developing children are knowledgeable, active, social human beings with personalities. They crave attention and activity. They have needs and desires, and they can attain many of them through their own skills. They can make most physical-world entities work for them. They have learned to use nonlinguistic communicative behaviors such as gestures to make other people attend to them and respond to their needs for certain physical objects and events. They also have learned to appreciate the warmth, security, and joy that comes from those cooperative and constructive interactions that are the hallmark of human societal living. Now they must take that final learning step into full membership in their human community—they must learn to use its spoken language. They must learn to use language because they have reached the limits of their abilities to live cooperatively and productively in their environment without it. Table 6–1 offers a review of the extensive nonlinguistic communication repertoire of children at about 1 year of age. As readers can see, the skills and the awarenesses that undergird communicative competence are well represented in infant's behavior. The only thing missing is the linguistic forms needed for true language.

It would appear that when adults observe such robust and skilled nonlanguage communicative abilities among children at this level of development, there is a shift in their expectations for their children. People around children at these developmental levels begin to expect more efficient ways of communication. They want and expect their children to become part of their verbal world. After all, they have taught their children a great deal about their physical and social environments and they have demonstrated time and time again that they will be cooperative

**Table 6–1**

Children's Nonverbal Communicative Repertoires at the Time They Begin to Use Spoken Language

| | |
|---|---|
| 1. High Rate of Contact Gesture Use | Extend object for *give* and *show*; take adult hand and place it on self or object; tug adult, arm or clothes |
| 2. High Rate of Distal Gestures | Finger point; extend open palm; wave bye-bye; shrug for "don't know" or "where?" |
| 3. High Rate of Pantomimic Gestures | Turn-on; take-off; unscrew top; open |
| 4. High rate of Intonated Vocalizations | |
| 5. Directs Communicative Acts Toward Partner | |
| 6. Waits for Response From Partner | |
| 7. Repeats Act if Response Is Not Forthcoming | |
| 8. Large Number of Intentions to Communicate | Desire for objects<br>Desire for actions<br>Desires for help<br>Desires for interaction<br>Desires for attention<br>Desire for recurrence (more, again)<br>Marks possession (mine, yours) |

and responsive to children's nonverbal communicative acts. They have helped them learn what many words mean and patiently modeled how they can be produced by the child. They have simplified their own language in ways that allowed children to discover what language forms and structures are needed and what they can be used for. Truly, it is time for children to take all of their knowledge and apply it to learning and using the language forms and structures they need to operate in their social environment. Fortunately, they are ready to do just that.

## STAGE I: SINGLE WORD UTTERANCES

The child's expressive use of language begins with the production of his or her first word along with his or her understanding that that word *refers* to some entity, event, or relationship in the environment. This attachment of linguistic forms to their referential *meaning* is referred to the *semantics* of language. The first symbolic speech event typically occurs between the ages of 10 and 14 months, but may appear a few months later even in normally developing children. With the appearance of the first word, the young child enters a period of one-word utterance production, which typically lasts for 4 to 6 months. Even though a child's utterances remain at one word for a period of time, the vocabulary used in these utterances will grow dramatically. It should also be noted that some "one-word" child utterances may actually be two or more words that were learned by the child as a single word, for example, "peek-a-boo," "Barney-book."

The use of single words as communicative acts provides an opportunity for an in-depth view of human language in all of its complexity. Although, the single-word speech act is the simplest *form* that oral language can take, it nevertheless reflects all of the elements and knowledge that human language requires to work. For example, one-word utterances are intentional acts, selected by the speaker in order to have some effect(s) that he or she desires. One-word utterances reflect language's use of *symbols* to *refer* to people, states, objects, events, and relationships. The word used in one-word utterances has been specifically selected by the speaker to *mean* a certain thing to a receiver—something that will evoke a desired response from that receiver. One-word utterances reflect the wide range of *knowledge* that a young child has about the world and the extensive vocabulary he or she has for expressing that knowledge. One-word utterances also reflect children's knowledge about the social world of people that they live in. It reflects their knowledge that other people are ready and willing to help them, to respond to their needs, and to teach them more about language as well as more about the ways of the world.

## The Vocabulary of One-word Utterances

As we have stressed, children's early words must be those that they can use to *refer* to the people, objects, actions, attributes, states, and relationships that make up their particular environment. Although young children's environments are generally rather similar, there are also many individual variations in them.

But, because all human beings find certain aspects of their environments particularly salient, and therefore important, the *general* nature of young children's earliest word vocabularies is rather similar. For example, children and adults alike are drawn to action events. Consequently, children seem to first learn to name objects that can be acted on, such as balls or toy cars, or things that can provide actions, such as radios or musical tops. They also learn the words to name the actions they see applied to objects. Words like "turn-on," "up," "push," and the old familiar "hit." For several months a child's interactions with adults have been focused on certain objects and situations and various kinds of actions on those objects and in those situations. Thus, individual children have specific knowledge and experiences that make certain words particularly appropriate and necessary for them.

If children are to be able to refer to the elements and aspects of their individual environments, they must have many different types of words in their repertoire. Bloom (1970) noted that the words in children's early one-word utterances, were of two types:

**1.** *Substantive forms*

**2.** *Functional or relational forms.*

According to her definitions, substantive words are those that "make reference to classes of objects and events that are discriminated on the basis of their perceptual features or attributes"; whereas function or relational words are those that "make reference to classes of objects and events of behavior that extend across such perceptually distinguished classes of objects and events" (p. 70).

*Substantive* words, then, are words that serve as labels for objects and actions in a child's world (e.g., "ball," "fall," "dada," "kitty," "jump," "kiss"). *Function* words are those that describe some relationship or state, which might apply to *any* of these objects or events, (e.g., "more," "all gone," "there," "more").

## Specific Examples of Children's First Words

We are going to look at three data displays that will help us to understand the general nature of children's earliest language forms. The first is Katherine Nelson's work in detailing and analyzing the first 50 words produced by each of 18 children between the ages of 12 and 24 months (Nelson, 1973). The source of the second and third displays of children's early words is provided by Lois Bloom's work identifying the major types of single words that she observed in her study of her daughter Allison's early language (Bloom, 1973).

Table 6–2 lists Nelson's analysis of children's first 50 words and includes a distinction between the percentages that occurred in the first 10 words and those that were observed in the first 50 words. It important to note that Nelson identified her word categories in terms of the child's intentions in using them, rather than translating them to conform to adult-level "form classes" such as nouns, verbs, and adjectives. This strategy causes us to focus on what children choose to *mean* in their early language. This perspective is important because it maintains our intent to be sensitive to how and why children use language rather than to become swept up into the more abstract notions about linguistics and grammar that tend to dominate our adult perspectives about words and language. As we will see, Bloom maintains the same child-focused perspectives in her data analyses.

On the basis of Nelson's data, it seems that the most common forms of early words is the "general nominal" (noun) and the next most common is the "specific nominal" (proper noun). Further, it can be seen that, as the child develops his or her vocabulary from 10 to 50 words, the relative proportion of *specific* nominals decreases, while *general* nominals increase. This means that children seem to name more of the generic things and events in the world and slow down in terms of adding more proper names or labels for specific, single-instance referents to their vocabulary. For example, they learned to refer not only to "Muffy," their own dog, but also to "doggies" in general.

In addition to the data on one-word forms provided by Nelson's study, Bloom's 1970 study, and her later analysis of one-word utterances produced by her daughter (Bloom, 1973) provide further insight into the nature of this level of language production. In all of this work, she identified the "meanings" of children's single-words by taking into account the immediate context in which they occurred. Like Nelson, Bloom maintained her focus on the *intentions* of, or *effects* desired by, the child producing the speech act. Only when the intentions of the child

**Table 6-2**

Summary of Nelson's Analysis of First 50 Words Produced by 18 Children

| Word Category | Example | % of first 10 words | % of first 50 words |
|---|---|---|---|
| I. Nominal—Specific (total) | | 24 | 14 |
|     People | "mommy" | | 12 |
|     Animals | "Dizzy" (name of pet) | | 1 |
|     Objects | "car" | | 1 |
| II. Nominals—General (total) | | 41 | 51 |
|     Objects | "ball" | | 31 |
|     Substances | "milk," "snow," | | 7 |
|     Animals and people | "doggie," "girl" | | 10 |
|     Letters and numbers | "e," "two," | | 1 |
|     Abstractions | "good," "birthday," | | 1 |
|     Pronouns | "he," "that" | | 3 |
| III. Action Words ( total) | | 16 | 13 |
|     Demand-descriptive | "go," "bye-bye," | | 11 |
|     Notice | "up," "look," "hi" | | 2 |
| IV. Modifiers (total) | | 8 | 9 |
|     Attributes | "go," "red," | | 1 |
|     States | "pretty," | | 6 |
|     Locatives | "hot," "dirty," | | 2 |
| | "all gone," | | |
| | "there," "outside," | | 1 |
|     Possessiveness | "mine" | | |
| V. Personal-Social (total) | | 5 | 8 |
|     Assertions | "no," "yes," "want," | | 4 |
|     Social-expressive | "please," "ouch" | | 4 |
| VI. Function words (total) | | 6 | 4 |
|     Questions | "what," "where" | | 2 |
|     Miscellaneous | "is," "to," "for" | | 2 |

*Source:* Data from Nelson (1973); table adapted from McLean and Snyder-McLean (1978).

could be determined, could the *meaning* of the single words uttered be identified with any confidence.

Bloom identified the same basic types of *substance* words that Nelson described—primarily *nouns*. She, noted, however, that her daughter initially used more *function* words in her earliest one-word utterances. Remember that function words are words that refer to relationships that can be applied *across* classes of objects, states, or events referenced by substance words.

We can gain an excellent feel for the kinds of words toddlers find important and useful by looking at Bloom's data. Table 6–3 lists the total *single-word utterances* produced by Bloom's daughter, Allison, at about 16 months. Table 6–4, which follows, offers the list of specific *function* words that Bloom observed in Allison's one-word utterances between 9 and 20 months of age.

An analysis of both types of word classes that children first use clearly reflects the objects, states, attributes, and events that children have come to recognize and understand through their months of interactions before language. They are words that refer to their particular environment and their unique experiences. In other words, these words that they first use *refer* to the games, the objects, and the action events that have been historically important to them and their interactive partners. Thus, again, children

**Table 6–3**

Single-Word Utterances and Their Frequency of Occurrence for Allison at 16 Months, 3 Weeks

| | | | |
|---|---|---|---|
| All gone | 1 | Mama | 9 |
| Away | 9 | Mess | 2 |
| Baby | 19 | More | 24 |
| Car | 2 | No | 21 |
| Chair | 14 | Oh | 3 |
| Cookie | 15 | Pig | 6 |
| Cow | 3 | Sit | 1 |
| Dada | 4 | Stop | 1 |
| Dirty | 2 | There | 30 |
| Down | 22 | Turn | 1 |
| Girl | 3 | Uh | 2 |
| Gone | 19 | Uh-oh | 7 |
| Here | 1 | Up | 27 |
| Horse | 1 | Wida | 1 |

*Source:* Adapted from Bloom (1973).

**Table 6–4**

Major Function Words and Their Apparent Meanings as One-Word Utterances

| General Relationship | Word | Function/Meaning |
|---|---|---|
| Existence | "there" | To point out objects |
| | "uh-oh" | To point out objects, particularly those that startled |
| Recurrence | " more" | First to request and later to comment on the recurrence of an activity or object |
| Disappearance | "away" | To comment on the disappearance of object which had existed in context |
| | "A' gone" | (Same as above) |
| Nonexistence | "no"$_2$ | To comment on nonexistence where existence had been expected |
| Cessation | "stop" | To comment on the cessation of an activity |
| Rejection | "no"$_1$ | To protest undesired action or comment on forbidden object (e.g., stove) |
| Action | "up"$_1$ | To request the action of being picked up |
| Location | "up"$_2$ | To comment on spatial location |

*Source:* Data from Bloom (1973); table adapted from McLean and Snyder-McLean (1978).

do not learn just to *name* things, they learn how to *refer to* the elements and events of the environment they have experienced and words that they know are also known by their communicative partners. This means that there is a constant pressure on children to learn the new words that refer to their new knowledge. For example, Bloom noted that her daughter added tremendously to her vocabulary of *substance* words as her communicative activities increased. This suggests that the *relationship* words needed in early conversations are somewhat finite, but that the demand for more and more substantive vocabulary words just grows and grows.

## *Knowledge* About the World
## Precedes *Language* About the World

As we have stressed previously, adult language users often reflect a perspective that children learn about their world by first learning words and then learning what objects and events these words refer to. As indicated in the discussion above, however, the opposite is more often true. The data from the research on children's early language (e.g., Bates, 1976; Bloom, 1970; Bloom, 1973; Nelson, 1973) indicated rather clearly that children learned to use language for coding what they *already knew* of the world of objects, events, and relations. While, of course, children will later gather much of their world knowledge from the language they hear, in these early months, they will depend first on their knowledge of the world to help them identify and learn the early words that they will first need to communicate in their unique environment.

Children have a wide range of knowledge about the various things in their environment. They know that these things differ from one another in various ways. They are aware of their perceptual attributes such as their relative size (*big, little*), and tactile properties (*hot, sticky, soft*). They also know that objects vary in terms of their functions. Some objects are to be used to eat, some to color pictures, and some to be manipulated so that they produce a certain object or sound. Children are also beginning to differentiate *states* of personal circumstances that can be referred to in ways that others can understand—states such as *hungry, sick, hot*. Children, at this point are also beginning to understand that, with language, they can *refer to* objects, events, and relationships that are not immediately present in the context of their conversations. Thus, they can choose to refer to something they desire in the future, something that they recall from the past, or something that they want but is missing (*all gone, no more*).

The notion that children first learn words and then learn their meanings was prevalent until the research findings of the 1970s. This perspective led to a period in which much of the remedial work offered to children with severe communication disabilities was focused on teaching words that the remedial specialists thought were important for the child to learn. After teaching such words through imitation procedures, it was thought that children would know, or quickly learn, the referents for the words they had learned to imitate. Instead, many, many children with severe disabilities such as severe mental retardation learned to say words that, at the time, they did not know the meaning of. As a result, although they often uttered these newly learned words, they used them inappropriately and, too often, with no clear notion about what their usage should bring about from their interactive partners. Today's remedial procedures are focused on teaching words that refer to objects, states, and event elements that young children with children with disabilities already know and that they *need* and *want* to be able to produce in their everyday interactive contexts. This is what parents and teachers of typically developing children do, and there is no reason to think that it is not also the best way to teach language to children with developmental language delays or serious disabilities. Parents and teachers alike, then, should always be helping young children to learn the words and phrases that they need to talk about the things that *they already know* about their world. Later, of course, we will teach new words in order to teach the child new concepts. But early on, we let the child's knowledge and communicative needs lead our language teaching.

## What Do Children *Do* With One-Word Utterances?

There has been a great deal of research on the *functions* or *uses* of children's early language. As we already know, these *functions* and *uses* are called the *pragmatics* of language. In fact, there are dozens of taxonomies that categorize such functions. Each listing takes a certain perspective from which to analyze these functions. Thus, each listing or taxonomy provides a slightly different view of them. To the nonspecialist in language, the often slight differences reflected in these taxonomies can be quite confusing. So rather than take you through a complex process of analyzing and comparing these several perspectives, we have chosen to offer one taxonomy, which we think best sets up a discussion of children's early language uses. John Dore (1975) observed a large sample of very young children's language utterances and analyzed the functions that he could identify by looking at the *utterance* itself, its social *context*, any additional actions or gestures made by the child, and the adult *responses* to these utterances. Table 6–5 shows the results of Dore's research as he identified what he called the *"primitive speech acts"* of young children. This

## Table 6-5
Dore's Primitive Speech Act Types

| Primitive Speech Act | Child's Utterances | Child's Nonlinguistic Behavior | Adult Response | Relevant Contextual Features |
|---|---|---|---|---|
| Labeling | Word | Attends to object or event; does not address adult; does not await response. | Most often none; occasional repetition of child's utterance. | Salient feature focused on by child; no change in situation. |
| Repeating | Word or prosodic pattern | Attends to adult utterance before his utterance; may not address adult; does not await response. | Most often none; occasional repetition of child's utterance. | Utterance focused on; no change in situation. |
| Answering | Word | Attends to adult utterance before his utterance; addresses adult. | Awaits child's response; after child's utterance, most often acknowledges response; may then perform action. | Utterance focused on; no change in situation unless child's response prompts adult reaction. |
| Requesting (action) | Word or prosodic pattern | Attends to object or event; addresses adult; awaits response; most often performs signaling gesture. | Performs action. | Salient feature focused on by child and adult; change in condition of object or child. |
| Requesting (answer) | Word | Addresses adult; awaits response; may make gestures regarding response. | Utters response. | No change in situation. |

*(continued)*

**Table 6–5**

*(continued)*

| Primitive Speech Act | Child's Utterances | Child's Nonlinguistic Behavior | Adult Response | Relevant Contextual Features |
|---|---|---|---|---|
| Calling | Word (with marked prosodic contour) | Addresses adult by uttering adult's name loudly; awaits response. | Responds by attending to child or answering child. | Before child's utterance, adult is some distance away; adult's orientation typically changes. |
| Greeting | Word | Attends to adult or object. | Returns a greeting utterance. | Speech event is initiated or ended. |
| Protesting | Word or marked prosodic pattern | Attends to adult; addresses adult; resists or denies adult's action. | Adult initiates speech event by performing an action the child does not like. | Adults' action is completed or child prevents action. |
| Practicing | Word or prosodic pattern | Attends to no specific object or event; does not address adult; does not await response. | No response. | No apparent aspects of context is relevant to utterance. |

*Source:* Data from Dore (1975); reprinted from McLean and Snyder-McLean (1978).

term reinforces the notion of language utterances as intentional *acts* of children on the people in their environment. Later in this chapter, we will show you how young children accomplish these desired functions by the words they learn, the phrases they construct, and the meanings that they communicate to others. For now, however, let's look at the details of the primitive speech acts that Dore identified in the language of very young children.

## A Closer Look at "Primitive Speech Acts"

**Requesting Action.** In many cases, children desire a specific action from a caregiver. They might want help. They might want a partner to continue a playful or constructive interaction. They might want a partner to provide an object for them. They might want the partner to stop an action he has been producing. They may want a partner to act on them or on some object in some certain way. They might want mother to provide more of a desired food they have been enjoying. Always, in this category, children want a partner to do something, but what they want them to do varies widely according to what the interactive episode is focused on and what the child wants to happen next. Clearly, however, the intention, or desired response, to the language act is predetermined by the child.

In these earliest stages of language use, young children are using one word to express their communicative intentions. At this stage, the context of the child's utterance, and any supplemental gestures or motor acts, are still important for comprehending what exactly the child intends. For example, if we simply list the *words* we hear a child utter, such as "ball," "cookie," "more," "on," and "dolly," we cannot interpret the child's intentions with much degree of certainty. If, however, we also have information about the context of the utterance and about the child's vocal inflection and we know the additional gestures or actions the child makes along with the word, we have a much higher probability of correctly interpreting his or her intentions in selecting the particular utterance produced. Look at the information below, and then interpret the intentions of the child.

I. Child holds out an empty hand toward mother and says, *ball.*

2. Child finishes eating a cookie, looks at Grandma and says, *cookie.*

3. Child holds out the music box that has run down, looks at daddy and says, *agin.*

4. Child gives brother a flashlight that they have been playing with and says, *on.*

5. Child looks in her bed, looks behind her, and then looks at mother and says *dolly?*

We can see that these words are not just names of things or actions, but rather are *acts* on another that have been chosen by the child to evoke a specific action from the communicative partner. And, when the context of the utterance is clear, so are the actions expected.

**Requesting Attention.** There are also many reasons for children to request the attention of their partners. They may do so to prepare a partner for an action they will be requesting. A child might request the attention of a partner only to share an interesting object or event, although some additional action usually follows such a request. Mothers constantly hear, "Mama" spoken rather emphatically by a child and accompanied by a pointing gesture. Sometimes a child may say "Daddy" to get his attention while he or she shows off a new skill. At other times, however, the child may be sharing a new object or event and wants his or her partner to demonstrate an action that is appropriate for some object, provide the object's name, or provide other information about it. By pointing to an unfamiliar person in the vicinity and uttering the word, "mamma?" a child might be asking his or her mother for reassurance in the face of some anxiety. In response, a mother might say, "Yes, that's Mr. Schultz, our neighbor. He's a nice man, isn't he? Say Hello." The partner's responses to requests for attention, like all other language function categories, are as many and varied as the interaction contexts that obtain between children and other people. As we will see later in this chapter, requesting, securing, and directing of the attention of other people are major and frequently used early language acts for young children. Many times these acts are preludes to requests for action to follow. Other times, the act is simply an end in itself, satisfied when mother says, "Yes, I see it."

**Answering.** Another function that children want to carry out with their language is to be *responsive* to their partners. One of the ways children can demonstrate their responsiveness to their partners is to answer questions that are put to them. Mother points to a picture in a book and says, "What is this?" Her child answers, "Kitty." On other occasions, mother might ask, "Where do you want to go?" ("Bye-Bye"); "Do you want another cookie?" ("Yes"); "What kind do you want—a graham cracker or an Oreo?" ("Oreo"); "Where does it hurt?" ("Tummy"). As you can see, within the act of answering, a child may be labeling objects, requesting action, requesting an object (e.g., an Oreo) , or providing information. This particular language act is also a prime example of doing two things simultaneously. We gave an example of such multiple uses earlier when we suggested that politeness terms were intended more to meet certain expectations of society than to express a specific desire of a speaker. Thus, when we say, "Please pass the salt," we are both expressing our intention as a speaker and meeting a societal rule. In the case of "answering," we are meeting an expectation of another person who has posed a question while at the same time, we are making reference to some meaning that we intend. Thus, this language act has referential meaning (a *semantic* relationship); a speaker intention (a *pragmatic* function), and a rule-meeting function (a *dyadic* function). These multiple functions will become clearer as we continue to examine the many uses of language.

**Requesting Answer.** Technically, of course, this category is part of the overall category of requesting action. However, it is such a specialized action request that most experts assign it to a category all its own. Because the action being requested is specifically a verbal one, it seems to deserve this separate recognition. A request for an answer is, essentially, a question. Questions have many linguistic structures in English. These structures usually involve more than one word. There is, however, one frequent dimension of a question that can be carried in one word, and that is its upward inflection. Thus, when a child says "bye-bye" with an upward inflection, his or her mother will more than likely take it as being a question and respond accordingly, "Yes, we're going bye-bye. We're going to go to the store."

The answers that children seek from others are as varied as any other broad category of language functions. In some cases, children may only be requesting a "yes" or "no" response to a request for approval or denial regarding some action that they want to take. In other cases, children may be seeking specific information from a care provider. In still other situations, a child may be seeking confirmation of a language act or other action. In a sense, the child is asking, "Is this the right word for that object?" "Is this what I should do with this object?" In a general sense, this category most often reflects a request for feedback from a partner. Clearly, this language function fits well with the notion that babies want to perform appropriately, constructively, and cooperatively in their interactions with others. They see their care providers as having the job of helping them to do so and the willingness to provide such help.

When children ask questions with their language, they expect an answer from their conversational partners. As children move into the two- and three-word stage, anyone who has spent time with young children is all too familiar with their frequent use of this function. From "What's that?" "Can I, Mommy ?" "Is it tomorrow yet?" "Are we there yet?" to "Where's daddy?" children seek answers that take many forms from requesting information to asking permission. Again, children understand the rules of human communication. They know that there is an obligation on the part of the partner to reply to such inquiries. In fact, they have come to understand that the obligation to answer questions is even a bit stronger than the obligation to respond to other forms of language acts. Thus, children quickly learn to use questions to increase the odds that they will get a response to something that might be, most basically, a simple request for action, for example, "Mommy, two cookies?" Mother answers, "No, but I guess you can have one more."

**Protest.** Children, like all humans, have many occasions to protest some action, statement, order, or request from the adults around them. They have already learned to protest with actions and gestures such as pushing mother's hand away, hitting at a sibling, or spitting out a food they dislike. Because these actions often evoke rather dire responses from caregivers, babies learn that protesting through language is slightly more acceptable. Thus, "No !" "Stop!" and "Don't" become frequent language acts for babies.

**Greeting.** Caregivers often start language instruction by following up with the verbal equivalents of some gestures that they teach babies early on. Thus, waving is supplemented with the words "bye-bye" and the word "hi" quickly follows. Babies come to understand that these salutations are part of the politeness rules for human interaction. Although not technically greetings, other politeness words such as "thank-you" and "please" are also included in most children's early language acts.

**Calling.** This is simply a specific type of request for attention or action from a partner who is not in the immediate vicinity or is not attending to the child. It might be used by children who are in some sort of distress and need action from a caregiver to help them out of the problem. Other times, it is simply meant to secure attention for the purpose of demonstrating something or sharing a new, particularly interesting event. A call to another person is specific and carries with it some direct urgency for attention or action. In a sense, a call is less polite than other requests are, and for this reason it carries a high degree of demand or expectation for a response from the partner called. It is interesting that when people show *less* politeness, we consider the language act to be more urgent and we react with added dispatch. The one problem with politeness acts is that they are time-consuming

### Some Primitive Speech Acts Are
### Not *Specifically* Communicative

As the reader can see, the language functions listed so far are directed to a receiver for the purpose of evoking some response. We have identified this action on other people as the *essence* of language. However, there are language utterances that are not specifically intended to have an effect on others. Speech acts of this type are intended to perform some act that the baby desires only for himself or herself. Since these types of speech acts are *egocentric* and perform some *private* function desired by the child, they carry no demand for a response from a listener. Dore identified three such functions among his listing and definitions of primitive speech acts.

**Labeling.** We often see children sitting in their room uttering the "names" of things. Dore observed these acts among children who were not aware of a receiver and seemed to be self-absorbed in this ritual. He surmised that this speech act was simply a type of exercise in which children were more or less "testing" their competence to *label* objects, actions, and/or events. I remember my early-talking older son crawling behind a rolling ball or another type toy, saying "ball, ball, ball" or "truck, truck, truck" seemingly oblivious that anyone was listening and, certainly, not looking for any response. It appears that children are simply checking their speech repertoire and applying it for their own enjoyment and satisfaction. In a sense the child might be asking, "Do I have the 'word' for this object? If so, I might as well use it."

**Repeating.** Young children often repeat a word or phrase they hear an adult use. There a number of different reasons why children do this. For example, in a videotape series we made several years ago, we had a scene in which 2-year-old Cindy was seated on a sofa with her daddy. She had a small necklace that she was trying to unhook so that she could put it around her neck. After many efforts, she handed the necklace to her father and said, "open." Her father responded to her request, and as he handed it back to her, he said, "There, it's *apart*." Cindy took the necklace, looked at it, and began saying *"a part, a part, apart."* Why she was doing this, we cannot be sure, but there are several possibilities. Perhaps this was a new word to Cindy, and she needed to try it out to see if she could produce it. On the other hand, many words are fun for children to say—they just "feel good." Listening to Cindy, I always felt that she simply enjoyed saying this word. Emphasizing different syllables on each successive utterance of the word, she just seemed to be having fun making this particular sequence of sounds. For the record, her father never did make a response to her utterance, and Cindy didn't seem to mind his ignoring of her speech act. It seemed clear that her "apart" was not directed to him.

We must remember that, when children are just beginning to talk, they are beginning the process of learning to produce thousands of words rather quickly. Although they have been babbling and making vocal noises for several months now, mastery of particular sequences of speech sounds is a whole new ball game. They must listen to the word and try to match the sound characteristics of the word. Sometimes they do very well. Other times, their speech development level might not allow them to be able to produce certain sounds or combinations of sounds. That's why, grandma becomes "*mamo*" and grandpa becomes "*paw paw.*" The speech sounds /m/ and /p/ plus the two vowels needed to produce these "approximations" are among the easiest English speech sounds for young children to produce.

We will look briefly at the development of the speech sounds children need to produce for their culture's particular language a bit later in this chapter. The point that we want to make here is that, in order to practice and learn these sounds, young children repeat many words and phrases that they hear adults use. Such practice helps their learning of new sounds, words, and phrases. It also allows them to simply have fun with what they have already learned to produce. We must remember that they are taking words that they have received auditorily and now trying to produce them themselves. As we can appreciate, this is a major task and one that requires children to monitor both the motor feelings of producing the word and also to listen to the product of their speech effort and compare it to the auditory model that they have heard produced by others. Some research indicates that people discriminate better between sounds that they have learned to produce than between sounds that they do not yet produce. A clear example is the difficulty most people have in understanding the words and phrasing in a language that is different from the one that they speak. Some languages use speech sounds that do *not* occur in other languages. Thus, when we hear sounds that do not occur in our language, we most often have difficulty understanding them. In the early stages of language development that we are discussing, children are working to learn to produce a mode of behavior that is *new* to them. The fact that it is an extremely complex behavior, with literally thousands of elements and combinations of these elements, should cause us to marvel at how readily they are able to make progress in acquiring it.

**Practicing.** Clearly related to *repeating* is the speech act of *practicing*. Again, this form of speech act is not usually a communicative act. It is simply an act that children produce for themselves to allow them to improve their speech and language skills. Practicing goes on throughout early childhood. Children playing "mother" or "teacher" with their dolls or other playmates are often "practicing" their skills at matching their language output with what they hear in the environments around them. As adults, we often find great humor in the ways that young children can adopt the vocabulary, tone, and phrasing of a "teacher" in their play. When we hear such accurate depictions of adult speech, we can see that children are not only learning words, but also the higher level nuances of different forms of adult speech. In a lecture I heard many years ago, Elaine Anderson, reporting on her research in sociolinguistics, reported that 5- to 6-year-old American boys, when asked to talk like a "Doctor," "routinely lowered their voice about 2 octaves and adopted a Viennese accent." "Ah," they might say in their lowest possible voice, "you are not feeling vell, eh? Vell, let's see vat is wrong wis you." For young children, learning language is, literally, practice, practice, practice. And how they enjoy becoming competent at talking like adults!

What we should take away from this review of the functions or uses of children's primitive speech acts is that they are selected by the *speaker* to effect some *intention* that he or she has. We should also be sensitive to the fact that, at this stage of one-word utterances, the intentions of the "speaker"might require a receiver to look at one or more of the language acts that preceded the one at hand. The receiver must also analyze the context and conditions in which an utterance is produced, including any nonverbal actions or gestures that the child produces. Without understanding all of the variables operating in the context in which a child's early, simple utterance is produced, we cannot begin to be sure that we fully understand the child's intentions in producing it.

We should also point out here, that Dore's list of speech acts lists some that are produced so that a speaker can meet some interaction rules that go beyond just his or her personal needs or desires. As we have seen, some utterances are produced in order to "answer" another person or to "be polite" in one's language exchange. "Please" or "thank you" are used to meet the desire of a speaker to follow the rules of social discourse. Of course, because these niceties in language work to increase the probability that a listener will respond to a speaker's request for attention or action, they do, indirectly, reflect back on the speaker's basic intentions in producing the language act in the first place. In other words, children learn that they are more apt to have their intentions responded to if they have "asked nicely."

# STAGE 2: TRANSITION TO TWO-WORD UTTERANCES

All of the research about the first words used by children emphasizes the difficulties encountered in being sure what the words children use actually mean to them. To make judgments about what children's utterances mean, we must analyze their words in light of the context in which they are uttered, any other child behaviors that accompany the utterance, and the best guess that we can make about apparent *responses or effects* that children expect as a result of the utterance they have produced. The ambiguity of one-word utterances points out the need for children to work to become less ambiguous by learning to produce utterances that carry their meanings more effectively and precisely. The need to improve their communicative effectiveness and efficiency led children to learn to use objects on their partners to better communicate their intentions, then to add gestures to their communicative acts, and then to learn to use speech in addition to gestures. All of these skill acquisitions by children allowed their receivers to better understand their utterances without needing to be in direct visual contact with the child.

Learning how to put more than one word together with others is children's next move in attaining more effective, efficient, and less ambiguous communication. When children can begin to refer to their topics in ways that reduce their partner's need to *interpret* all of the variables involved in the context in which the utterance is produced, the demands on their partner are greatly reduced, and the child's feelings of competence are greatly increased. When language utterances are finally effective enough to be *freed* from their immediate context and still be understood, communicative effectiveness has just taken another major step as a truly skilled human behavior. Let's look at how this move happens.

As we have examined children's progress through the many stages of language development, we can see that the process is a gradual one, one in which each new skill level includes and builds on the one preceding it. Thus, children do not just move into entirely new language skills and types. Rather, they improve their current skill level by adding a new skill that improves their ability to communicate more efficiently and effectively. Thus, each stage of a child's development is marked by the emergence of a major new skill in his or her production of spoken language. Nothing makes this point better than the child's move from one-word utterances to multiword utterances. In fact, if we examine this move in some detail, we can see the kinds of small steps that are involved in a child's progress.

Children do not just jump from the use of one-word utterances to the use of multiword utterances. Rather, research by Bloom (1973) showed that, on the way to true multiword utterances, they first enter a stage where every now and then, they utter two, *one-word* utterances very close together. Although the practical effect is a two-word utterance, the reality is that children are simply cojoining two, one-word utterances to attain the "meaning" of their utterance. After some experience with these so-called, "successive one-word utterances," children discover the ability to produce more complex meanings by constructing utterances that truly combine two words to carry the desired meaning. At this point in their development, children are still intent on "meaning" certain things to their communicative partners. They are ignorant of the *grammar* of a language. They have no real rules to follow to put two words together, so they seem to come up with some logical ways to help themselves produce meaningful two-word utterances. Three prominent strategies seem to be reflected in two-word structures in early child language. Although no one can say for sure that any of these posited strategies accurately describes what children are actually thinking, they do seem to offer plausible explanations of many of the two-word utterances children produce. The first is a strategy of a *Topic-Comment* word order. The second is a strategy of using a *Pivot-word* + an *x word*. The third strategy that seems possible is simply expressing the words they want to use in the *temporal* order in which they occur in the real-life event they are referring to. We will look at each of these possible strategies in more detail.

## Topic-Comment Constructions

Chomsky indicated that the child's first evidence of a beginning grammar is children's common tendency to structure their utterances by referring to the *topic* of their utterance and then making a *comment* about that topic (Chomsky, 1965). This is not an unreasonable strategy for a child to use, considering that, at this stage, a child is usually geared to identify the "common focus" that is present in the context of his or her utterance. Thus, if the common focus in an interaction involves a kitten, a child might say something like, "Kitty, meow." To which an adult might respond by *expanding* the utterance, "Yes, that's right. The kitty says 'meow.'" Remember, adults most often use complete sentences even when conversing with very young children. Therefore, such expansions come naturally to them. Other such "Topic-Comment" combinations seem rather typical for child utterances. "Cookie, more" ("Is that cookie all gone? OK. Here is some more cookie.") "Daddy, work" ("Yes, daddy's at work. He should be home for dinner.") "Head hurt" ("Oh your head hurts? Show me where it hurts.") "Truck big." ("Yes that is a big truck. It is a big red truck"). Notice that these utterances seem to be readily understood by adults. Notice, too, how all of their typical expansions offer the child models of the correct English syntax for the *meaning* the child is expressing.

The same thing happens with adult *emendations* (corrections). For example, a child, using the topic-comment strategy might say, "Lipstick Mommy" and her parent might respond, "Yes, that's mommy's lipstick," demonstrating that the possessive relationship is marked *before* the object is named. Similarly, the child might say, "All gone milk" and the adult emends the utterance, "Is your milk all gone? Well, maybe we can find more milk. Say, 'My milk is all gone. More milk please.'"

## Pivot word + X word

Research also indicates that many early childhood utterances reflect a strategy of using a certain *pivot* word, paired with any one of a large number of substance words to complete the utterance (Bloom, 1973). A good example of this strategy can be heard when children take a certain *function* word, and follow it with many other words. For example, a child might use "no" as a *pivot* word and produce such utterances as:

"No milk"

"No dolly"

"No medicine"

"No all gone"

The interesting thing is that all of these identical syntactic structures can feature a different meaning of "no." In the first case, it might mean "milk is nonexistent." The second utterance might be heard when a child is role-playing the admonishment of her doll for some pretend transgression. The third usage might be used as a rejection of a medicine being offered by mother. And the final utterance might be a form of double negative in which a child means that her cookie is *not* all gone.

While other function words such as "more," "there," and "this" are frequently observed in pivot word + *x*-word constructions, some *substantive* words can also serve as pivot words in such constructions. "Mommy" is an example. A child might be heard to use *Mommy* in identical utterance structures to refer to several different *semantic grammatical* roles, for example, *agent* of an action, the *receiver* of an object, an *attribute* of an object, or a *possessor* of an object.

"Mommy push" (Mommy as agent of action)

"Mommy apple" (Mommy as receiver of object)

"Mommy sock" (Mommy as attribute of sock, i.e., describing a pair of nylon stockings)

"Mommy lipstick" (Mommy as possessor of lipstick)

## Chain Words in Their Real-World Temporal Order

A third strategy children seem to use when putting words together is simply marking the order in which referents occur in the real-world event. We have noted that children are drawn to action events. In real life, action events unfold in a temporal order. A batter swings, he hits the ball, and the ball goes into the air toward the outfield. A child, wanting to refer to a sequence such as this, then, might say, "hit ball" or "ball gone." In much later stages of development children who are still unable to put four and five words together and say, "The man hit the ball a long way in the air," might, however, segment the utterance into a series of two-word phrases, for example, "Man hit," "hit ball," "ball all gone."

There are other relationships that reflect a temporal order and children seem comfortable using that fact to string words together. In fact, many child *Topic-Comment* utterances seem to reflect temporal factors, for example, "Daddy bye-bye," "Mommy drink," "blocks fall 'gin."

In all of these early strategies for constructing two-word utterances prior to any real sense of grammar, the *expansions* and *emendations* that come from adults in response to such utterances teach children how to produce their desired meanings in more complete and accurate utterance structures. Thus, by using their language as best they can in these early, simple structures, children evoke all kinds of good language models from adults. These models show children complete sentences with the correct grammatical positioning of the words needed to express the meaning the *child* wants to express. The latter point is an important one. *The best way to be successful in teaching very young children better language skills is to help them to say what they want to say in semantically accurate and grammatically correct ways.*

## STAGE 3: VOCABULARY GROWTH AND THE DEVELOPMENT OF TWO- AND THREE-WORD GRAMMATICAL UTTERANCES

### Vocabulary Growth in the Toddler Stage

Parents are frequently amazed at the words their toddlers can use. This amazement extends both to the number of words used, to the *kinds* of words that children begin to utter as they approach 2 years of age. Once children begin talking, their vocabulary grows by leaps and bounds. Carey (1978) reported that vocabulary grows at the rate of about five words per day from 18 months to 6 years. Throughout this period, many children have the ability to relate a new word to its referent after only *one exposure* in a phenomenon called "fast mapping" (Carey, 1978; Dollaghan, 1985; Nelson, 1973).

Children apply many strategies in relating a new word to a referent. For example, if an unknown word is used by an adult, a child might scan the context of the utterance and select the one "new" object or action that is present in that context and assume that it is the referent for the new word. Similarly, if a child has a red block and a yellow block and knows the color red, when mother asks for the yellow block, the child ignores the known red block and picks up the nonred, yellow block. By *exclusion* of the known color, then, a new color referent is established. This strategy of exclusion allows children to make use of the words and referent relationships that they already know to help them figure out new entities, actions, and relationships that occur in the context of their interactions with mature language users. Of course, children are not always correct in their deductions, so their adult partner is there to correct and refine the word-referent relationships. Children depend on this feedback from their communication partners. As we have stressed throughout this book, the *context* of these vocabulary learning interactions is very important. If new words are introduced, it helps the child greatly if the referent of the new word is prominent in the context in which it is used. Adults routinely spend a great deal of effort in making sure that they offer conditions in which new word-referent relationships are taught clearly. They contrast words. For example, "This bunny is *soft*, this block is *hard*. This is *big*, this is *little*. This is *mine*, that is *yours*." Children even request help in learning new words, "What dis Mommy?" Sometimes they ask more indirectly. Holding up a glass, a child may say "cup?" Mother replies, "No that's not a 'cup,' that's a 'glass,' see it has no handle." "Glass—no cup" replies the child.

The process of vocabulary teaching is so pervasive in our interactive environments, that it becomes automatic for children to "fast map" and for parents and other adults to teach and contrast new and old words. Of course, constant refinements and expansions of one's vocabulary continue through a lifetime.

Let's think about some of the meanings that we see as important to young children who are first using their language to play their roles in interactive scenarios with people who are important to them. We have emphasized the point that knowledge about the environment precedes the language needed to refer to the environment. Think back to our discussion in Chapter 5 about the kinds of knowledge that children acquire before they learn language. Think of the sensory motor concept of *causality* and realize that it is this concept that sets up the knowledge of action events that have segments that relate to *agents*, *actions*, and *receivers* of actions. Think of the *object concept* that allows children to realize that, even if an object is out of sight, it can still exist and, therefore sets up the notions of lost, recurring, and/or located somewhere else. Think of the concept of *means-ends* that allows children to understand that they have the means to attain desired goals. They can push, pull, put in, take out, and so on. Think of the thousands of objects that they have manipulated, put together, or put into one another.

When you have recalled these details of children's early knowledge holdings, you can see that, indeed, the words and meanings that children begin to use with their partners *refer to* entities, states, events, and relationships that they already know. Remember, too, that all humans tend to find the same aspects of the world interesting and compelling. Action events are important to everyone. They reflect our dynamic environment and children must know how to talk about them and their component elements of *agents, actions,* and *objects.* Children find many occasions in which they need to refer to the *locations* of items ("doggie house"), the *recurrence* of items ("more cookie"), the *disappearance* of entities ("milk all gone"), and the *recurrence* of action by the *agent* of that action ("daddy, more up"). Also very important in these early utterances are the *perceptual attributes* of objects ("big doggie," " long stick," "pretty, shiny star") as well as the *sensory attributes* of entities, ("sticky candy," " soft bunny," "hot pan"). One can see why children must learn new vocabulary items rapidly!

## Learning to Put Words Together Grammatically

As children's vocabularies increase and the things they need to "mean" become more complex, they are faced with the challenge of stringing their words together in a way that assures that all of their potential new intended meanings are accomplished. The old, simple strategies of topic-comment, pivot-open, and simple temporal order will not work for the more complex meanings a child now has to express. Children are beginning to understand that there are rules for putting words together in the right order. This means that they must begin to acquire these rules for stringing words together in longer and longer phrases. As adults, we refer to these rules as the *grammar* of a language, and we codify them in an abstract linguistic system called the *syntax* of a language. We call such a system *abstract*, because it describes these rules in a way that can be applied to any utterance, regardless of meaning. For example, a syntactic rule of English describes a simple declarative sentence as a "Noun phrase" plus a "verb phrase," and we might detail one such structure as "Article + noun + verb + article + adjective + noun." Thus, "The boy ate the chocolate-chip cookie" or "The girl dressed the Barbie doll."

In children's early language, however, the first "syntax" children learn is derived, not from the abstract adult grammar rule system, but rather from the rules children learn about "how to mean" certain things. For example, English-speaking children have learned that, if you are going to describe an action on something, the *agent* of that action is named first, then the *action* is specified, and then the *object* of the action is indicated. Thus, "Boy hit ball." Rather than an abstract grammar such as *noun + verb + noun*, a child's word-ordering rule system seems to be a semantic grammar of *agent* of the action, + the particular *action* carried out + the *object* of the action, or "who did what to whom?"

Obviously, children don't learn the rules about how to arrange the words in utterances immediately. As with all aspects of their development, children must work through a series of large and small learning steps to finally arrive at a consistent and accurate grammar for their early language. The adult strategies for helping children learn language are still present in adult-child interactions and continue to be crucial in this stage. Adult *responsiveness* to children's utterances, their teaching strategies of *expanding* their utterances, and their gentle corrections of children through *emending* of their utterances are all prominent in this process of the development of a grammar in early childhood.

After weeks and months of adult expansions and emendations of child utterances, children's language efforts reflect the effects of such adult strategies. They move from simple, topic-comment structures to more advanced, semantic grammar constructions such as the *agent + action + object, attribute + object,* or *object + location* constructions, which reflect a better understanding of the correct grammatical positioning of words. These better grammatical structures reflect children's learning of some simple rules for talking about the important entities, relationships, and states in their environment. Their utterances might still be simple, two- or three-word phrases, but they are grammatical and, importantly, they are consistent in the way they express certain meanings. Table 6–6 offers an expanded listing, description, and examples of this stage of children's language development. You can see in this table the rules by which children structure their utterances in ways that allow them to talk about certain entities, states, and relationships that are important in their environment. The first column shows the *meanings* that children find important to talk about. The middle column shows the formal *syntactic*

**Table 6–6**

Typical Grammatical Utterance Types at About 18 Months of Age

| Semantic Structure | Syntactic Structure | Example |
|---|---|---|
| **Two-Word Utterances** | | |
| 1. Agent -action | Noun + verb | "Eve read" |
| 2. Action-object | Verb + noun | "Read book" |
| 3. Demonstrative entity | | "That book" |
| Nomination | that/it/etc., + noun | "It book" |
| Notice | hi/see/etc., + noun | "Hi belt" |
| 4. Possessor—possession | Noun + noun | "Mommy lipstick" |
| 5. Entity-attribute: | Verb + more | "Fall 'gin" |
| Recurrence | More + noun | "More milk" |
| Nonexistence | No/all gone + noun | "No doggie" "All gone milk" |
| Attribute | Adjective + noun | "Big train" |
| 6. Entity—locative | Noun + noun | "Sweater chair" |
| 7. Action—locative | Verb + noun | "Sit chair" |
| 8. Agent—object | Noun + noun | "Mommy sock" |
| 9. Conjunction | Noun + noun | "Umbrella boot" |
| **Three-Word Utterances** | | |
| 1. Agent-action-object | Noun + verb + noun | "Mommy spill juice" |
| 2. Agent-action-location | Noun + verb + noun | "Daddy sit chair" |
| 3. Action-object-locative | Noun + noun + noun | "Throw ball here" |
| 4. Agent-object-locative | Noun + noun + noun | "Daddy ball chair" |

*Sources:* Data from Brown (1973), Bloom (1970), MacDonald and Blott (1974); table adapted from McLean and Snyder-McLean (1978).

makeup of the utterance. The last column offers an example of each type of utterance.

## CHILDREN MOVE ON TO MORE MATURE GRAMMARS

Once children have learned a repertoire of basic grammatical rules for meaning various things, they are quite understandable to adults and to each other. And they are well on their way to acquiring a language that reflects the full grammar of their language. There is, of course, much more to learn, but the rudiments are there. Obviously, children have learned literally thousands of words to talk about both their existing and their newly developing knowledge. They are also learning to produce more mature phrase structures. For almost a year now, children have been producing one-, two-, and three-word phrases made of, primarily, just the major words needed for the utterance they intend. Because of this use of just the few major words in their early utterances, children's early speech is often described as *telegraphic*, reminiscent of the abbreviated messages that were used in telegrams (e.g., "Arrive Tuesday. TWA Flight 464. Meet me."). To better meet their communicative needs (and their receivers' ever-increasing demands), children must also now move into more traditional language structures by lengthening their phrases and adding all of the "little" words that they have been leaving out of their first, short phrases. In the year between 24 and 36 months of age, typically developing children do just that. They develop tremendous vocabularies; they refine their articulation of speech sounds; and they acquire grammar that is closer to the mature and correct grammar expected of mature language users. They still talk about things that children talk about, but they do so with a relatively complete repertoire of skills in constructing understandable, polite, and effective utterances.

### Acquiring the Little Words of Language

As we noted above, one thing that children need to do to be able attain a higher level of grammar is to learn the "little" words that are important to their specific language. The little words are important to every language. In English, they include *determiners* like *a/an, the, this,* and *that.* They are also *prepositions* like *in, at, by, to,* and *with.* These are sometimes called *function words* because they tend more to do things that make our language work, rather than express a substantive, "dictionary" meaning. Yet it is these little words that will extend children's ability to produce the longer phrases and sentences needed to carry their communicative meaning.

These little words are not the ones pictured in children's books. Rather, they are words that are truly learned in the context of using language. This means that children must listen carefully to the language being spoken around them and begin to learn the prepositions, articles, auxiliaries, and pronouns of that language. The article *the* doesn't really "mean" anything, and prepositions such as *of, on, in,* and *from* require a great deal of exposure before children can figure out exactly what they mean. Similarly, the use of pronouns such as *he, she, them,* and *they* to replace proper nouns require time for the child to understand. The adult strategies of *expanding* and *emending* children's utterances provide the children with examples of how we use these little words. Using these adult examples, children imitate these little words and use them in their phrases long before they truly understand them. In this stage where children are refining their language and producing longer phrases, they learn to imitate many complete adult phrases without understanding what some of the words mean. Then, when they try to use these words on their own, they depend on the feedback from adults to tell them if their usage is correct. For example, a child might say, "Her hit me" only to be given the correct form by an adult, "*She* hit you? Well, we'll have to talk to *her* and tell *her* that we don't do that here." Now a child might have a better understanding of *she,* but what's this *her* stuff? As you can see, it's really quite a task for a child to attain a full understanding of his or her full language system.

It is only later in their formal education programs that children will learn about determiners, pronouns, prepositions, and adjectives. They will not formally parse a sentence until middle school. Yet, for the most part, young people will have been speaking in meaningful, grammatically correct, sentences for many years. Once again, it seems a truism to say that children have learned language "by doing." They have used it to do things for themselves. If they have used it incorrectly, there are natural consequences and learning opportunities that allow them to improve their language skills. Educators of young children should take special note of this point. For many years professionals in many disciplines attempted to teach better language to children by teaching predetermined language repertoires. In other words, they have taught what *they* (the professionals) thought children should learn. In addition, too often, they taught it in the abstract. That is, they taught *vocabulary and utterance structure*, rather than teaching children how to say what they wanted to say. Now, it seems clear that language learning in the early years should be carried out as it is in the natural home teaching environment—by setting up contexts for truly using language. These teaching contexts can be carefully planned and structured "joint action routines" (Snyder-McLean, Solomonson, McLean, & Sack, 1984) that allow teachers and clinicians to target the language forms that seem appropriate for the individual children in their groups. These structured teaching contexts reflect the need for *real* language to do *real* things. In this sense, a working educational environment is truly ideal for teaching "real" language. We will be talking more about this when we look briefly at treatment options in Chapter 7.

### Grammatical Morphemes

As if having to learn all of these little *words* isn't enough, children at this stage must also begin to learn the functions of certain single speech sounds and small clusters of sounds, which are often *not* words but affect meanings in their language. These groups of sounds are called *grammatical morphemes* and, like function words, they carry meanings that are important in a language. These morphemes (meaning units) are usually added to other words to carry some additional meaning that is important to the language system being used. These important morphemes can take the form of complete words or just parts of words (suffixes and prefixes).

A full discussion of the types and functions of grammatical morphemes is beyond the scope of this book and the needs of its readers. But we do need to have a general understanding of what morphemes are and what they do in our language. Perhaps the best way to understand grammatical morphemes is to look at a list of some of them and to examine what they are used for in a language. Table 6–7 offers Brown's list of the earliest morphemes learned by children, in the typical order in which they are learned by most children, and gives examples of each (Brown, 1973).

As you can see from Table 6–7, these morphemes serve important functions, as they help a speaker follow the *rules* of a given language to express specific meanings, and shades of meaning. They allow us to add small meaning units to existing words to indicate such things as plurality, past tense, contractions, and possessives. They include many of the "little" words that we have already discussed. You can also see that the acquisition of all of these small, but extremely important, aspects of the language takes children some time. Several of the listed verb forms are not acquired until about age 5.

### Table 6–7
Brown's 14 Grammatical Morphemes and Their Order of Acquisition

| Order of Acquisition | Morpheme | Specific Form(s) |
| --- | --- | --- |
| 1 | Present progressive | -ing |
| 2–3 | Prepositions | in, on |
| 4 | Plural (regular) | -s, -es, etc. |
| 5 | Past irregular | came, ran, etc. |
| 6 | Possessive | -'s |
| 7 | Uncontractible copula | is, am, are (as in: "She is pretty") |
| 8 | Articles | a, the |
| 9 | Past regular | -d, -ed, -/t/ |
| 10 | Third person regular | -s, -/z/, etc. (as in: "She runs") |
| 11 | Third person irregular | does, has (as in: "They do" vs. "She does") |
| 12 | Uncontractible auxiliary | is, am, are (as in: "They are running") |
| 13 | Contractible copula | -'s, 'm, 're, (e.g., "She's pretty") |
| 14 | Contractible auxiliary | -'s, 'm, '-re (e.g., "They're running") |

*Source:* Data in columns 1 and 2 are from Brown (1973); table adapted from McLean and Snyder-McLean (1978).

Between 3 and 4 years of age, typically developing children are able to produce well formed, declarative sentences with generally appropriate grammar. They are able to use grammatical morphemes and meet the requirements of the English language for hundreds of rules that govern its use. For example, they begin to make sure that their verbs and nouns agree as to plurality or singularity; they begin to use auxiliary verbs when needed, and they pretty well know the most important irregular verb forms. They can ask simple questions using *wh*-words, such as *what*, *where*, and that favorite of children, *why*. Obviously, they still make many grammatical errors, but they seek corrections and "fast map" in this domain, just as they did in vocabulary learning. Language teaching at home continues, but is now supplemented by formal educational experiences. And learning to read will loom large in their continuing language learning process. Reading will allow them to better understand their grammar, add to their vocabularies, and add greatly to their knowledge about the world. Their language skills have attained their full range of functions, and children are now full members of their human society. Skilled in that society's most unique and productive behavioral system—its language.

## STAGE 5: THE FINAL REFINEMENTS IN EARLY CHILD LANGUAGE: SENTENCE TRANSFORMATIONS, DISCOURSE RULES, AND SPEECH SOUND MASTERY

There are, of course, many more things about language that children need to learn before they attain the mature level of language usage that is expected from adults. Although any in-depth analysis of this further learning gets us into levels of linguistic study that are beyond the scope of this book, we will look at three more advanced language skills. These final skills are ones you will see children beginning to grapple with between 3 and 5 years of age.

### Sentence Transformations

To this point, even with addition of function words and grammatical morphemes, most child utterances are still straight *declar-*

*ative* sentence forms. Future learning will allow children to alter these declarative structures to produce interrogative forms in which part of the verb phrase is shifted from the middle to the beginning of a sentence, for example, "*Are* you going to school?" It will also allow transformations to imperative forms such as, "Stop doing that!"; subjunctive sentences such as, "If I were you, I wouldn't do that"; and even more complex interrogative forms using auxiliaries such as, "Would you let me go first?"

All adults will be called on to help children in their pursuit of the complexities that we know language must be able to handle if people are to be socially successful. All of these transformations are described in the grammar rules of our language that children will study formally in high school. But, as adults, we will be involved in helping children construct these transformations many years before that.

## Discourse Rules

Another skill that children will be pursuing beyond the preschool years is learning how to take their proper roles in *conversation*. We may have children communicating with language, but we are still a long way from having them *converse* with us with any degree of mature effectiveness or social appropriateness. Earlier in this book, we discussed the child's learning of two important conversational skills: turn waiting and turn taking. But, of course, much more is involved in good conversation, and it is not terribly complex. It is, however, important enough that adults get involved in teaching some rudimentary conversational skills to children quite early in their language development years. There are basic rules that we seem to concentrate on with children who are beginning to use language in interactions with other language users:

1. Respond to the *linguistic content* of your communicative partner's utterance. Young children often forget that they have an obligation to listen to their partner's utterance and respond to it appropriately and pertinently.

2. Maintain or add to your partner's topic; or if you change the topic, you must note your awareness of the fact that

you did not follow the rules. Children are great at topic shifts, for example, "Do you understand why you must do better at keeping your room picked up?" "O.K. Mamma, Bobby got a new train set. Can I go to Bobby's to play. Can I?" Of course, we must allow children this freedom to introduce their own topics, but they need to understand that we are granting them a privilege.

3. Provide enough information in your utterance to be *effective* in your communication. Children often keep their topic or focus a secret with utterances such as, "Mama, You know that guy? Well, we all know he did it." What guy? Who's we? Who's he? Did what?

4. Don't provide so much information that you are not *efficient* in your communication. We have all heard a child's description of some TV episode that ends up with the child providing every line of dialogue. As we have noted, once children get your attention, they often want to keep it, and keep it, and keep it. Obviously, we can't allow such abuse of the rules of turn taking in conversation.

5. Be polite. Say please, thank you, and excuse me. Don't interrupt. Such niceties seem to be a lost cause in today's world and we feel it. The interesting and important awareness is that such politeness has always been a priority in the language teaching of young children in almost all cultures.

Adults begin teaching these conversation rules early. Children get so excited and enamored with using their language that they often violate these rules. However, these conversational rules become more and more important as children reach school age. Adults insist on relatively effective, efficient, and polite communicative acts from children. We know that language is critical in shaping adult judgments about children. We also know that good language and proper conversational skills are the eventual hallmark of a considerate and educated person. We want our children to attain such status. Such preparation starts way back with "peek-a-boo" and "my turn-your turn."

# THE DEVELOPMENT OF THE SPEECH SOUNDS OF A LANGUAGE

As readers can see, the final stages of language development among very young children begin to make heavy demands on the abilities of the children to produce their spoken language with some precision. One of the most demanding levels of precision comes at the level of accurately producing the speech sounds of a language. If the meaningful sound units of a language cannot be produced in ways that others can understand them, communication is severely compromised. In this discussion of the final stages of language learning during the early childhood developmental phases, we need to take a brief look at the speech sounds of English and understand what they demand of the child.

Any spoken language is made up of a finite set of single sounds that are strung together to produce utterances that have meaning in that language. Standard spoken English, for example, is produced by stringing together 25 consonant sounds, 12 vowels, and 6 diphthongs. Many of these sounds are quite simple in their articulation and are easily produced by babies learning to talk. Other sounds, however, require rapid, complex movements and precise placements of the tongue. Because educators regularly encounter children who have not yet mastered the sounds of their language, it is important for them to understand the rudiments of the sound system. There is generally a logic to children's articulation problems, but it takes some awareness of the nature of a language's sound system to see that logic and to understand what kind of a problem is present. Although we will not attempt to make our readers experts in the phonology of English, we think it will be helpful to examine the nature of this system of English speech sounds.

## How to Get the Most Out of this Section

The material covered here might seem complex to readers who have not studied language and speech in any real depth. It really isn't as difficult as it might first seem. One thing that will help readers understand the information presented over the next few pages is to produce the sounds being discussed. If readers will say the sounds as they are mentioned and, at the same time, watch their production in a mirror so they can see the movements of the tongue and its placement in their mouth, this discussion will be much clearer. Placing a finger in front of the mouth and your thumb on your throat will allow you to feel the airstream produced by a speech sound as well as the presence of voicing or unvoicing. Looking into a mirror as you produce various sounds will allow you to observe the placement of the tongue on many of them. These observations will provide the reader with first-hand information about the details of speech articulation. So, rather than let yourself be limited to the material on the printed page, you should analyze your own production of speech sounds as you read this section. If you will produce all of the sounds as we describe them, and examine your actions while doing so, the information in this section should be quite clear.

## The Speech Sounds of English

Table 6–8 offers a list of the 43 speech sounds used to produce the English language. These sound families are called *phonemes* and are defined by the fact that they make a difference in *meaning* in the language. Very simply, the contrast between the words *sit, fit, lit,* and *kit* show that /s/, /f/, /l/, and /k/ are all phonemes of English because, when they occur in similar sound combinations, the words they produce mean different things. Similar contrasts of what are called minimal pairs, for example, *sit/fit, man/tan, fate/fake, fit/feet* demonstrate that the other consonants and vowels sounds identified as phonemes of English can meet the same type of test. That is, with all other factors being equal, each of the phonemes listed makes a difference in meaning.

We say that the phonemes of English are sound "families" because many of the sounds vary in their form when produced in running speech. For example, the /t/ in *take* is different from the /t/ in *fat* because the /t/ in take has a little puff of air at its end, while the /t/ in fat does not—at least the way most people say it. These sounds are, however, both heard as /t/ in our language. In fact, there are other slight variations of the phoneme /t/ that are used in English. It is important, however, for a speaker of English to be within the overall boundaries of these sound

**Table 6–8**
The Phonemes of English

| Consonants | | Vowels | Diphthongs |
|---|---|---|---|
| /p/ peep | /v/ veal | /i/ beet | /ai/ buy |
| /b/ bib | /s/ sun | /ɪ/ bit | /au/ bow |
| /m/ my | /z/ zone | /e/ say | /oi/ boy |
| /t/ toot | /š/ shoe | /ɛ/ set | |
| /d/ deed | /č/ chop | /æ/ sat | |
| /n/ noon | /ž/ azure | /a/ far | |
| /k/ cook | /ǰ/ judge | /ɔ̆/ up | |
| /g/ gig | /r/ rear | /u/ mood | |
| /ŋ/ singer | /l/ lull | /ʊ/ pull | |
| /θ/ ether | /h/ hail | /o/ obey | |
| /ð/ either | /w/ wail | /ɔ/ fall | |
| /f/ fife | /y/ you | /ɚ/ burr | |

families if he or she is to be readily understood by other speakers of English.

## Types of Speech Sounds

English speech sounds are of three different types, namely, *vowels, consonants,* and *diphthongs.* We need to understand the differences in these different types of sounds.

### Vowels

These are simple sounds that are created by placing the tongue in certain positions in the mouth and sending vocalizations to resonate in the mouth. The vowel /i/ as in beet is made with the tongue placed high in the front of the mouth. The /u/ as in boot with the tongue high and in the back of the mouth. Other vowels have different tongue positions. Say each of them yourself and look into a mirror to see the tongue take its position for the vowel you intend to produce.

## Diphthongs

These sounds are basically two vowels uttered one right after the other. Thus, they also are formed by tongue placements. In a diphthong, the tongue position will shift. Say the diphthong /oi/ (*oil*) and watch in the mirror as the mouth opens and the tongue goes back and low in the mouth for the /o/ vowel and then closes with the tongue moving high and to the front of the mouth for the /i/.

## Consonants

These sounds are just the opposite of vowels. Rather than being simple vocalizations with the tongue in a certain position, consonants create different kinds of *constrictions* or *interruptions* of the breath stream and, in that way, produce sets of very distinctive sounds.

These *sets* of sounds reflect some interesting characteristics. For one thing, these various sets of sounds are developed in ways that minimize the number of different things a speaker must learn. For example, although English has 24 different consonant sounds, these sounds are related, so that speakers only need to learn to make sounds in six *manners*; using seven different *places* in the mouth where the airsteam is constricted in order to produce them. *Voicing* is used with 15 sounds, while *no-voicing* occurs with 9 of them.

This matrix of consonant differences is shown later in Table 6–9. But before we look at this matrix, let's examine the elements that we will see in it. We shall see, for example, that there are six ways that we produce consonant sounds in English. We call these ways, the *manners of articulation*. They are listed and described below:

## Manners of Articulation

*Stops* [/p/, /b/, /t/, /d/, /k/, /g/]—In *stops*, the airstream directed into the mouth is stopped completely, and then is exploded to produce the sound.

*Fricatives* [/f/, /v/, /θ/, /ð/, /s/, /z/, / š/, / ž/, /h/]—In *fricatives*, a very narrow constriction is created by placing the tongue in contact with certain parts of the mouth structure. The air is then forced through this stricture and produces a friction noise.

*Affricates* [ /č/, /ǰ/ ]—*Affricates* are a combination of stops and fricatives. The airstream is stopped and exploded through the stricture created for either / š/ or /ž/.

*Oral resonants* [ /l/, /r/]—*Resonants* have a vowellike quality in that they are produced by sending the voiced airstream into a mouth cavity created by placement of the tongue in a certain configuration. In the /l/ the air passes around the sides of a tongue that is elevated in the mouth. In the /r/ the tongue is elevated quite high in the mouth and the voiced air stream is directed into the cavity.

*Nasal resonants* [/m/,/n/, /ŋ/]—Nasals are produced when the soft palate is lowered and air is allowed to enter the nasal cavity. Different sounds are produced by different shapes of the oral cavity.

*Glides* [ /w/, /y/]—*Glides* are produced by starting with one vowel and then gliding into another vowel. For example, the /y/ in *you* starts with the tongue high and front, making the /i/ as in *eat* and then gliding into the /u/.

### Places of Articulation

When we examined the six *manners* of articulation, we saw that we have several different sounds listed for most of them. This is because each of these manners can be executed at a different place in the mouth. For example, among the *stops*, we produce the /p/ by stopping the air by closing the lips tightly and then exploding it, whereas the /t/ is produced by stopping the air with the tongue placed against the gum ridge and exploding it from that place. Thus, within each manner, there are sounds that are produced at different places in the mouth. The seven *places of articulation* in which sounds are produced are identified across the top of the matrix shown in Table 6–9. These are labeled as follows:

*Bilabial* [/p/, /b/, /w/, /m/]: Lips are together

*Labiodental* [/f/, /v/]: Lower lip is placed against the upper incisors

*Lingua-dental* [/θ/, /ð/]: Tongue tip to upper incisors

*Lingual-alveolar* [/t/, /d/, /s/, /z/, /l/, /n/]: Front of tongue placed against the alveolar ridge (gum ridge)

*Lingual-palatal* [/š/, /ž/, /č/, /ǰ/, /ř/]: Tongue front placed on the front part of the hard palate (back from the alveolar ridge)

*Lingua-velar* [ /k/, /g/, /ŋ/]: Back of tongue to soft palate

*Glottal* [ /h/]: The *glottis* is the opening between the vocal folds in the larynx. In producing the /h/ in *hot,* air is forced through the open, but tensed vocal folds.

## Voicing

You have probably noticed by now that there is one more contrast between many consonants. Many consonants are produced with *voicing* and others are produced with *no voicing.* For example, both the /s/ and the /z/ are produced in the same *manner* (fricative), and in the same *place* (lingual-alveolar). However, the /s/ is unvoiced while the /z/ is *voiced.* The contrast between *voiced* (VD) and *unvoiced* or *voiceless* (VL) sounds when they occur are marked along the side of the matrix, immediately under the *manner* classifications. These contrasts are also shown in Table 6–9.

### Table 6-9
Consonants of English by Manner of Articulation and Place of Articulation

| | Bilabial | Labio-dental | Lingua-dental | Lingua-aveolar | Lingua-palatal | Lingua-velar | Glottal |
|---|---|---|---|---|---|---|---|
| *STOPS* | | | | | | | |
| Voiceless | p | | | t | | k | |
| Voiced | b | | | d | | g | |
| *FRICATIVES* | | | | | | | |
| Voiceless | | f | θ | s | š | | h |
| Voiced | | v | ð | z | ž | | |
| *AFFRICATES* | | | | | | | |
| Voiceless | | | | | č | | |
| Voiced | | | | | ǰ | | |
| *RESONANTS* | | | l | | r | | |
| *NASALS* | m | | | n | | ŋ | |
| *GLIDES* | | | | | y | w | |

## Developmental Errors in Articulation Among Young Children

There are some typical errors that young children make as they learn to produce the sounds of their language. We will briefly examine three of them.

### Substitutions

Children often simply use a sound they know in place of one that they have not yet mastered. This usually happens among sounds that are related to one another in *manner* of articulation but differ in the *place* of articulation. For example, if a child has learned the *fricative* /f/, he or she will often substitute it for the /θ/, which is also a fricative but is produced in a different place, e.g., the /f/ is a labio-dental. while the /θ/ is a lingua-dental. These sounds are both unvoiced and their acoustic properties are very similar. Thus, when a child says *fumb* instead of *thumb* or *teef* for *teeth* it doesn't cause adults too much trouble. Similar substitutions within *manner* (or manners that are very similar) include: /s/ for /š/; /w/ for /l/ ; /θ/ for /s/ (a lisp).

When substitutions occur across *manners*, however, comprehension in usually more severely affected. If, for example, a child substitutes a /t/ for a /s/ (a stop for a fricative) and says "I taw tat," (I saw cat) comprehension is more likely to be affected, especially in running speech.

### Omissions

Many times, young children will simply omit sounds, particularly in multisyllable words. In early speech, this is the way children simplify speech so that they can tackle it. Thus, *grandma* becomes *gama* and *tomorrow* becomes *mara*. Later, however, in more mature, running speech, omissions can cause serious problems in comprehension.

### Distortions

Sometimes, particularly in vowels and vowel-like sounds such as resonants, children simply do not get their tongues placed correctly and, consequently, do not produce a sound correctly. A child distorts /r/ or /l/ for example, and gets words that are close to *wun* for *run* or *wike* for *like*. These distortions are relatively benign in a child's early years. If they continue into later childhood and adulthood, however, they often affect comprehension and result in speech that sounds immature or babylike.

The reader can see that speech sound articulation is a rather complex, but organized system. Obviously, there are many things that can go wrong. Obviously, too, it takes a child some time to learn all of its nuances. Fortunately, however, unless there are serious motor or neurological problems, disordered sound systems are quite amenable to treatment. Usually, children require careful instruction on how to produce various sounds and intense training to help them replace the incorrect productions with the correct ones. A competent speech-language pathologist will have many strategies and methods for carrying out this task successfully.

## PREVIEW: IN SUCH A COMPLEX PROCESS, THINGS CAN GO WRONG

Clearly, the structural design and the power of the human brain makes such complex learning possible. Just as clear, however, is the fact that children's acquisition of the language that prevails in their culture must be guided, modeled, and rewarded by others around them who know the language. In this book, we have attempted to portray this complex process of teaching and learning. Because our experience with young children has shown us that not all children acquire a full and correct language system, we know that this process sometimes fails. It is important, then, to look at what can go wrong in the process and what can be done to ease the effects of such a failure. In the final chapter of this book, we will examine this topic.

## SUMMARY

- Around 1 year of age, typically developing children can communicate effectively and extensively *without* language, but with the acquisition and use of one-word utterances, they are able to communicate a wider range of intentions.

- At roughly 18 months of age, children acquire richer vocabularies and begin producing two- and three-word utterances that reflect word orders that are consistent and approximate true grammatical forms.

- At 2 years of age, children begin to extend their telegraphic utterances into more typical phrases and sentences that contain the little words of language, such as articles and prepositions.

- At 3 years of age, grammatical morphemes begin to emerge, reflecting children's true understanding of many of the grammatical demands of their language.

- Also at 3 years of age, children begin to demonstrate the final refinements of sentence transformations, conversation skills, and speech sound development that will complete their attainment of a rich and effective language system.

## References

Bates, E. (1976). *Language and content.* New York: Academic Press.

Bloom, L. (1970). *Language development: Form and function in emerging grammars.* Cambridge, MA: MIT Press.

Bloom, L. (1973). *One word at a time: The use of single word utterances before syntax.* The Hague: Mouton.

Braun, R. (1973). *A first language in the early stages.* Cambridge, MA: Harvard University Press.

Carey, S. (1978). The child as word learner. In M. Halle, J. Bresnan, & G. Miller (Eds.), *Linguistic theory and psychological reality* (pp. 264–293). Cambridge, MA: MIT Press.

Chomsky, N. (1965). *Aspects of a theory of syntax.* Cambridge, MA: MIT Press.

Dollaghan, C. (1985). Child meets word: "Fast mapping in preschool children." *Journal of Speech and Hearing Research, 23,* 449–454.

Dore, J. (1975). Holophrases, speech acts, and language universals. *Journal of Child Language, 2,* 21–40.

MacDonald, J. D., & Blott, J. P. (1974). Environmental language intervention: A rationale for diagnostic and training strategy through rules, context, and generalization. *Journal of Speech and Hearing Disorders, 39,* 244–256.

McLean, J., & Snyder-McLean, L. (1978). *A transactional approach to early language training: Derivation of a model system.* Columbus, OH: Charles E. Merrill.

Nelson, K. (1973). Structure and strategy in learning to talk. *Monographs of the Society for Research in Child Development, 38*(149).

Snyder-McLean, L., Solomonson, B., McLean, J., & Sack, S. (1984). Structuring joint action routines: A strategy for facilitating communication and language development in the classroom. *Seminars in Speech and Language, 5,* 213–228.

# 7

# DELAYS AND DISORDERS IN THE LANGUAGE DEVELOPMENT PROCESS

# WHAT CAN GO WRONG, AND WHAT WE CAN DO

## LEE K. McLEAN

## Key Concepts

✔ Any factor that seriously interferes with the strategies used by children to learn or adults to teach communication and language skills will interfere with the child's acquisition of speech and language.

✔ Problems with the acquisition of language are described as either language delays or specific language impairments.

✔ Problems with the acquisition of the production of language (speech) are described as either articulation disorders or fluency disorders.

> ✔ Early identification and, especially, early intervention yield the most effective results in the treatment of language disorders.
>
> ✔ The more you know about *how* children learn language, the better prepared you will be to support language learning in all of the children you interact with every day.

## INTRODUCTION

At the beginning of this book we stressed that a typical child's development of communication and language was a *sensible* process. We think that we have demonstrated this point by describing the processes of teaching and learning that begin with a helpless but alert and stimulation-seeking newborn interacting with an environment rich with interesting physical entities and supportive and responsive adults. We have seen that all of these interactive experiences between babies and their physical and social environments typically produce an orderly process of motor, cognitive, and social learning that are eventually combined to produce both human communicative behavior and, eventually, a symbolic linguistic system that we call language.

Although this overall process is *logical,* we must also recognize that it is a *complex* process and that, as in any complex process, things do not always follow a typical course. It is encouraging to realize, however, that the overall process of early childhood learning is somewhat *overdesigned* and, therefore, can sustain some inadequacies in any one, or even several, of its elements and still produce development and learning that is at least adequate. It really takes some major disruptions in the process to cause *severe* problems in a baby's broad learning patterns. However, deficiencies in children's development in any of the important learning domains (including language) *do* occur and the more we understand about how and why these deficiencies come about, the better we will understand what can be done to enhance or fully correct some of them.

Thus, in this chapter we offer a broad view of the kinds of problems that can occur among a wide population of young children. We will also look at the resources that can be enlisted to focus on the possible causes and treatment of these problems. Educators, parents, and other persons who are in regular and sustained contact with young children often are the first people to recognize problems among young children. Thus, it is important for them to be aware of the nature of some typical problems that can occur in the developmental processes and, importantly, what can be done to secure early help for children with problems. Early recognition and early treatment of children's developmental problems, including their acquisition of communication and language, can be quite successful. Thus, it is critical for professionals who are in a position to secure early evaluations and treatment for children suspected of having problems to do so. Hopefully, what you have learned about the developmental process and the acquisition of language from this course of study will help you to take action in cases where children need help.

This final chapter, then, is designed to provide educators and others who deal with very young children with the perspectives that will help them decide to refer children for expert assessment and treatment in any number of developmental and learning domains—but particularly in communication and language.

In the first six chapters of this book, we focused on how typically developing infants and young children learn their culture's language system. We have noted that *most* parents and *most* children do just fine in the language teaching and learning process. However, most is not all. Statistics from the National Institutes of Health and the U.S. Department of Education tell us that the most common developmental problems in early childhood are those involving the development of speech and language abilities. Approximately one out of every 10 preschool children experiences problems in learning to produce speech correctly; and about five children out of every 100 will have significant language delays or disabilities (Office of Scientific and Health Reports, 1988).

## NATURE AND CAUSES OF EARLY SPEECH/LANGUAGE DISORDERS

Many developmental speech and language problems are so subtle that they do not evoke concern from adults who are not attuned to the speech and language skills of typically developing young children. A 4-year-old child may be producing his or her speech sounds in ways that are perfectly normal for 2-year-old children. A 2-year-old may communicate very effectively with gestures, but not speak any words. Or a 3-year-old may be speaking words, but not yet using the early grammar and syntax that we expect of most 3-year-olds. Children with these mild delays or disorders often respond well to early treatment programs that provide enhanced stimulation and instruction specifically focused on the areas in which their development is lagging.

There is, however, a small percentage of children (approximately 1 to 2%) who have speech and language problems that are not so mild. In the most severe cases are children who have *no* speech or language systems at all. Indeed, there are children who have not yet discovered how to communicate intentions, even by simple gestures. Such severe communication and language disabilities usually occur in children who have pervasive cognitive, neurological, or physical disabilities. These severe disorders or deficits in speech and language will require intensive treatment programs involving professionals from many disciplines.

It is not difficult to understand why language delays and disorders are so common in young children when we consider the complex of factors involved in all of the early knowledge that children must acquire as they develop to the point of being able to successfully master language. In earlier chapters, we identified the many things that typically developing infants and toddlers do that contribute to their learning to function socially and to communicate their intentions and desires to others. We described these child contributions as their "acquisition strategies." We also described the responsiveness and support that caregivers provide to help children to discover both thing skills and people skills. When these teaching repertoires were applied to communication and language learning we referred to them as adults' "facilitation strategies." It is no surprise then, that any factor that seriously interferes with the development and use of either these child learning or adult teaching strategies will also interfere with the child's successful acquisition of his or her culture's speech and language system. Let's look generally at the conditions that can interfere with these systems in the critical early stages of language development.

## Factors that Interfere With
## Children's Acquisition Strategies

In Chapter 4, we discussed many ways that typically developing infants and toddlers respond to people and things in their environments; and we noted how these response tendencies, or "strategies," help young children learn their culture's language system. You will recall that these strategies include attending and responding to other people, attending to the common focus of interactions, trying to act on and have some effects on both the people and things in the environment, listening selectively to speech that is directed to the child, selectively imitating certain words or phrases in that speech, and producing plenty of communication and speech for other people to respond to.

Of course, the inborn tendency to respond to the environment in these ways is a function of the infant's brain and neurological system, which allow the newborn to perceive and process environmental stimuli and to respond and learn from them. It is the infant's brain and neurological system that allow the child to emotionally attach to other people and to see, hear, touch, feel, explore, experiment, and learn from these environmental experiences. And, it is the continuing growth of this system, the building of millions of new neural networks, that allow the child to integrate what he or she has learned and thus continue to learn and develop new skills.

We know, then, that anything that damages or interferes with the development of an infant's overall neurological system has the potential of jeopardizing his or her motor, cognitive, communicative, or linguistic development. We also know that such damage can be caused by a large number of prenatal (before birth), perinatal (during the birth process), or postnatal (after birth) insults to the developing infant. Prenatally, one major influence is the child's genetic code. There is strong evidence that certain speech and language disorders may be hereditary, that is, they may be carried in a gene that can be passed from parent to child. Although we do not know the specific hereditary mechanism for all of these disorders, we do know, for example, that certain types of mental retardation, neurological disorders, and speech and language disorders tend to run in families. Some speech and language disorders (e.g., stuttering) also tend to be more common in boys than in girls, suggesting that a sex-linked gene may be associated with these disorders. In addition to inherited genes, specific genes can also be damaged or lost at the time of conception. A well-recognized example of this is Down syndrome, which is most often the result of an extra chromosome that attaches to the 21st pair of chromosomes at the time of conception. This chromosome, and the genetic material it carries, is then reproduced in all of the new baby's cells, causing the baby to develop the features and characteristics of Down syndrome.

Beyond genetic causes, a number of other prenatal factors related to the mother's health and well-being can influence the unborn child's developing brain and neurological system. One of these factors is poor nutrition. If the pregnant mother's diet does not contain adequate nutrients, vitamins, and minerals, she cannot provide these essential building blocks to her unborn baby. Alternatively, if the mother is ingesting other substances (including alcohol, prescription drugs, or illegal, "street" drugs), these will be absorbed into the unborn infant's fragile, developing neurological system. Of course, serious illness or trauma to the pregnant mother can also cause damage to an unborn infant's neurological system.

There are additional risks to the newborn's neurological system during birth (perinatal risks) and in the early months following birth (postnatal risks). Perinatally, the greatest risk is anything that interrupts the supply of oxygen to the infant's brain before he or she is able to breathe air on his or her own. This risk is greatest in the cases of very difficult or very premature births. Following birth, the newborn's brain and central nervous system will continue to develop for several years. During this period of infancy and early childhood, the child's neurological system is particularly vulnerable to insults. Physical trauma to the infant's head or neck at this stage can result in permanent brain damage. This is why it is so dangerous to shake children, especially very young children.

Illnesses in a child's early years can also result in brain damage. Lead poisoning, seizures associated with high fevers, or infections affecting the brain or central nervous system (encephalitis) are examples of early childhood illnesses that can result in permanent brain damage. A very common childhood illness, fluid and infection in the middle ear (otitis media), has even been shown to contribute to delayed language development, because the temporary hearing loss that accompanies it can cause disruptions in language comprehension and production at critical periods in a child's development. Consequently, if middle ear infections are chronic in the child's early months, serious disruptions of communicative development can occur.

It is important to remember here that factors that interefere with the development or functioning of the brain can have highly specific effects on a child's ability to acquire different aspects of language learning. Some brain damage can affect the fine motor abilities of the phonation or articulatory mechanisms needed to produce sounds and running speech. Injuries to other parts of a child's brain may prevent that child from being able to *comprehend* speech. Still other insults may damage the ability to *formulate* speech and language messages.

Clearly, then, many pre-, peri-, or postnatal factors can have a direct, negative impact on the child's overall learning abilities and, thus, on his or her language development. For this reason, children who have any one of a wide array of neurological disabilities, including serious motor problems, vision or hearing impairments, or mild to moderate levels of mental retardation, will almost always show the effects of these impairments in both the learning that *prepares* infants for language learning and in the linguistic development process itself. Truly serious conditions such as severe autism or severe mental retardation usually result in rather global developmental problems that have devastating effects on the development of both speech and language. Children with such pervasive neurological disruptions to their development and learning will almost always need some expert help to compensate for the ways their disabilities limit their acquisition of the broad range of knowledge that they need to acquire communication and language.

## Factors that Can Interfere With Caregivers' Facilitation Strategies

In Chapters 2 and 3, we discussed the many ways that mothers, fathers, and other caregivers help young children learn their language system. You will recall that these caregiver "facilitation" strategies include establishing and maintaining joint attention and joint actions with the child; establishing interactive, turn-taking routines with the child; responding to the apparent intent of the child's communicative behaviors (movements, vocalizations, facial expressions, gestures, and words); talking to the child about things that are in the here and now; using simplified language forms, or "parentese," when talking to the child; expanding and emending the child's utterances; and, perhaps most important of all, encouraging and rewarding the child's own efforts at talking.

We have seen that these caregiver facilitation strategies are complementary to the infant's own language acquisition strategies, creating effective language teaching-learning partnerships between young children and their caregivers. Fortunately, most parents, adults, and even older children will adopt these strategies, without even thinking about it, whenever they interact with infants or young children. However, there are exceptions, and when a child's primary caregivers and communication partners do not provide this type of support for a child's learning, that child is at serious risk for language delay or disability.

Let's consider the factors that might interfere with caregivers' providing effective language learning environments for their children. All of our adult facilitation strategies require that the mature communication partner is able to focus attention on the young child and is motivated to establish and maintain an interaction with that child. Drawing on our own experiences, we can all think of times when we would not meet these requirements—times when we were too busy, too distracted, or too sick to even think about interacting with an infant or toddler. Unfortunately, some caregivers are chronically too busy, too distracted, or too sick to focus their attention and energies on a young child.

Any condition that produces serious and constant stress in the caregiver's life can jeopardize his or her ability to provide a supportive language learning environment. These stress factors can include major illness, drug or alcohol addiction, poverty, or mental health problems. In a day-care setting, simply having too many very young children, and too few caregivers, can also create this type of stress. Finally, some young parents lack the maturity to focus on the infant's needs and wants, because they are still absorbed in their own needs. These can include very young parents or parents with mental retardation or mental illness.

The reader will have realized, by now, that many of these factors that can limit caregiver facilitation strategies can be exacerbated by poverty. In this country, communities with very high rates of poverty also tend to have high rates of substance abuse, mental illness, and teenage parenting. In this light, it is sobering to consider what we know about the number of young children in this country who are growing up in poverty. Recent data tell us that one in four, or 25%, of America's young children live in poverty today, and half of those children live in homes that fall below the legal definition of *extreme* poverty. Further, in some states, the poverty rate for young children is nearly double these national averages.[1]

These statistics are alarming to all professionals who work with young children. For those of us concerned with children's language development, these numbers are especially disturbing in view of results from a recent study of children's language development in the first 4 years of life.[2] In this study, researchers compared the early language environments and language skills developed by children growing up in homes with different income levels. They found that children growing up in poverty heard fewer words and fewer encouragements for talking than did children in middle class homes. The children from poor homes also heard many more negative commands ("Stop," "Don't do that," etc.) in those early years. By the age of 3 years, children living in poverty had significantly smaller vocabularies and lower IQs than the middle-class children. Further, the same researchers found that the differences in early language experience were the most significant factors related to these lower scores. The same early experiences were also significantly related to lower language abilities at 9 and 10 years of age.

These findings, combined with what we know about the number of children growing up in poverty today, suggest that one in four of America's young children is at real risk for failure

[1] Data on child poverty rates taken from the National Center for Children in Poverty (Columbia School of Public Health) newsletter, *News and Issues*, Winter 1996–1997, Vol. 6, No. 2 , and are based on the center's 1996 report, *One in Four: America's Youngest Poor.*

[2] This research is reported in the 1995 book, *Meaningful Differences in the Everyday Experience of Young American Children* by Betty Hart and Todd Risley. (Paul Brookes Publishing, Baltimore, MD.)

to develop the language skills they will need for success in school and in adult life. On a more encouraging note, these data also suggest that providing high-quality language environments in children's early months and years can make a big difference in their future language development. For this reason, it is very important that all professionals who interact with young children, particularly those growing up in poverty, understand how language develops and how carefully developed programs of enhanced early experiences can support that development.

Among young children being raised in poverty, one group that seems to be at particularly high risk for school failure is children whose home language is not standard English. This group includes children from non–English-speaking families who have recently immigrated to this country. In all parts of the country today, young children enter public school speaking a great diversity of languages, including Spanish, Vietnamese, Laotian, Serbo-Croatian, and many, many others.

This group also includes children whose families speak a regional or cultural English dialect that differs in specific aspects of its pronunciation or grammar rules from the dialect known as Standard English (SE). In America, there are a number of such dialects, including Appalachian English (AE), southern English, and Spanish-influenced English. Certainly, the dialect that has received the greatest public attention in recent years is the African-American dialect, identified by some organizations as Black English (BE) and by others as Ebonics. All of these dialects have their own grammar rules and distinctive vocabularies and are highly valued and productive within the communities in which they are used (American Speech-Language-Hearing Association Joint Subcommittee of the Executive Board on English Language Proficiency, 1998). However, children whose families speak a non-English language or a nonstandard English dialect at home will face the challenge of having to learn Standard English as a second language in order to succeed in school and, often, in their chosen careers or professions.

It is important here to stress that poverty does not necessarily equate with ethnicity. There are many people of every race or ethnic background who live in poverty. It is also important to stress that poverty does not equate solely with a lack of money. Indeed, there are many kinds of "capital" and money is only one of them. For people of any ethnic background or heritage, a lifetime living in poverty has effects on many aspects of that person's capital holdings. Often, intellectual capital has been diminished by a lack of education. Often, too, the emotional capital among parents in poverty has been compromised by the need to work in dead-end jobs or the need to continue for years and years on social welfare programs. The maintenance of intact families also seems to be difficult in conditions of extreme poverty. A single mother working two jobs most often will not have the time nor energy to provide the quality interaction that guarantees that her child will receive the benefits of optimum "facilitation strategies" on her part. Poverty also limits the availability of toys, books, and recreational experiences, which are important to the learning of a rich language system. This litany on the negative effects of poverty could go on and on. But most professionals studying this book probably long ago arrived at the conclusion that the ideal and "typical" developmental processes that we have described are severely compromised in conditions of extreme poverty.

Despite all of these problems, most children developing in poverty *will* acquire a functional language system. Research indicates that this system may differ, both qualitatively and quantitatively, from the language abilities of children raised in middle-class economic conditions. But it is apparent that the drive of neurologically intact children to acquire a system of socially needed communication skills cannot be completely disrupted by conditions of poor social nurture. The language developed by children raised in extreme poverty or social isolation may be limited, but it is usually adequate to function in the home environment. The drive to acquire language is truly among the more robust of human drives. Remember what language means to the quality of human life; and it makes sense that it takes so much to seriously threaten its development.

## Interaction of Child and Environmental Factors

To this point, we have focused on risk factors that can affect either the child's acquisition strategies or the caregiver's facilitation strategies. Finally, it is important to note that these factors can and do interact with each other. For example, a premature infant will have a neurological system that is not yet fully developed. This factor, in itself, would pose some risk to the child's language development. However, that risk can be overcome by caregivers who are able to learn and use specific strategies for interacting with their baby. Alternatively, if the infant's caregivers, or caregiver, are under significant stress due to poverty or any of the other stressors we identified above, these two risk factors will interact with and compound one another. As this cycle continues, the infant's delayed development and other problems related to his or her prematurity may add further to the parent's stress and further weaken the parent's ability to provide an effective language learning environment.

In discussing the ways in which infants affect and are affected by their environments, Arnold Samaroff (1975) described this as a "transactional process." Thus, when both the child and the caregiver bring risk factors to their partnership, the impact on the child's development is more than just the sum of these risk factors; it is multiplied and exacerbated by this transactional process of mutual influence. Figure 7–1 illustrates this transactional process.

The schematic model in Figure 7–1 illustrates the circular nature of human interactions and communication. An infant's initial act provides an antecedent condition that evokes some response from the caregiver. The caregiver's response then provides both a consequence to the infant's act and an antecedent condition for another act from the infant. This give-and-take, "transactional" pattern characterizes all human interaction and is important in the context of this chapter because it shows that less than adequate responding on one partner's part necessarily has effects on the nature and quality of the other partner's behavior. Thus, a child who does not bring a full set of acquisition skills to this partnership will not reinforce an adult's facilitation behaviors, and *vice versa*. Quite simply, if either the adult or child doesn't play his or her part in these early interactions, the quality of the other partner's efforts will suffer negative effects. Thus, the poor responsiveness of a child with developmental delays will often extinguish the efforts needed from the adults around him or her. We have stressed throughout this book that both adults and children "fine-tune" their behaviors to each other's level. By doing so, in cases of typical development, each partner "drives" the other partner to new and usually higher levels. Such an escalating spiral on both sides of the dyad is critical to the entire

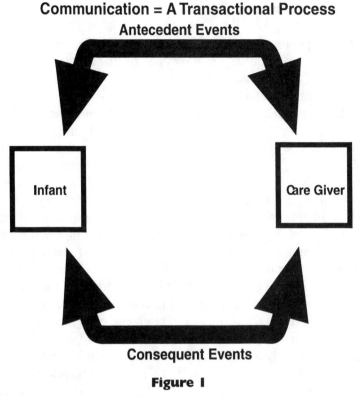

Figure 1

The Transactional Process

process of development. When this escalation fails to occur on either side of the partnership, real trouble looms.

Having reviewed and enumerated all of these risk factors, it is important to remember that the vast majority of children develop speech and language quite normally. Human infants are innately predisposed to learn language and mature speakers are equally predisposed to help them in that learning. Thus, despite great individual differences in parenting styles and resources and tremendous variation in child learning styles and opportunities, only one child in 10 will show any significant delays or problems in this critical aspect of development. The remainder of this chapter focuses on children who have some type of speech or language disorder. We will begin by describing the specific types of disorders that children might exhibit.

## Language Disorders

Generally, professionals who specialize in childhood language disorders distinguish two major types of disorder: *language delay* and *specific language impairment.* As we noted earlier, any risk factor or disability that affects a child's cognitive, motor, and/or social development is also likely to affect that child's language development. In many of these cases, the child simply develops receptive and expressive language more slowly than other children. When a child is significantly slower than other children in language development, that child will be diagnosed as having a *language delay.* In many cases, these language delays are relatively mild. A 3-year-old may understand and use language structures more typical of 2-year-olds; or a 2-year-old may understand single words, but not simple phrases, and may be just starting to produce words. For these children, a short period of early intervention is often effective in completely overcoming the initial delay.

At the other extreme, a few children with severe cognitive or neurological disabilities may be so delayed that they do not develop any real receptive or expressive language during the preschool years. Early intervention for these children is also very important and effective—but, it often will not eliminate the child's delay completely. Until recently, children with no expressive language were simply identified as being *"nonverbal,"* and were often not considered candidates for communication intervention services. However, major advances over the past decade have greatly changed the outlook for these children. Improvements in computer technology have allowed the design of portable communication devices that can produce speech output for children who can not produce speech themselves. In addition, research has shown that there are important differences among these so-called "nonverbal" children, reflecting their attainment of different milestones in the development of prelinguistic, intentional, and conventional communication (McLean, McLean, Brady, & Etter, 1991). Understanding these important differences allows us to design more appropriate and effective treatment programs for these children.

As you will recall from earlier chapters, the first of these major milestones is the child's discovery that she can affect other people through her communication acts. This discovery is the key to the child's progression from preintentional to intentional communication. For children who are not yet demonstrating any intentional communication, treatment will begin with helping the child to develop very basic social interaction skills, including some form of intentional communication. Other nonverbal children do communicate intentionally, but use a very limited set of behaviors and simple gestures to communicate only their most basic wants and needs to other people. For these children, treatment will initially focus on expanding the range of communication meanings and forms that the child can use. Still other nonverbal children will use a relatively sophisticated set of conventional gestures, and even intonated vocalizations, to communicate a wide array of meanings and intentions to their communication partners. For this last group of children, treatment will typically focus on helping the child learn to use a more effective, symbolic communication system, often in a mode other than speech.

The other major type of early childhood language disorder is, in some ways, more complex (and more perplexing) than the general language delay. This is the disorder identified as a *specific language impairment* (SLI). The generally accepted definition of SLI is a significant language delay (at least 12 months below the child's mental age) in a child who has a normal IQ and does not have any significant hearing impairment, behavior or emotional problems, or neurological disorders (Stark & Tallal, 1981). The exact nature of SLI varies from child to child. In some children, only expressive language seems to be affected; others show disorders of both receptive and expressive language. Further, the severity of these impairments varies greatly. Many children will have a delay only in the emergence of spoken words or the use of specific grammatical forms (e.g., appropriate use of auxiliary verbs, tense markers, etc.) and/or sentence structures (e.g., main verb clauses). Other children may have very severe language learning disabilities that persist throughout the child's school years and significantly impact both academic and social success.

## Speech Disorders

Children who are successful in attaining a spoken language system may, nevertheless, have serious problems in their overall communicative efforts because their speech production deviates from "normal" speech. Speech disorders affect the child's production of language, rather than the language itself. The two major types of speech disorders that we find in young children are *artic-ulation disorders* and *fluency disorders*. Communication disorders in which speech sounds are distorted, omitted, added, or substituted inappropriately are defined as articulation disorders by the American Speech-Language-Hearing Association (ASHA, 1993).

As we noted earlier, very young children make many types of predictable articulation errors that are a normal part of speech development. These predictable errors result in the types of immature speech that we expect from toddlers (e.g., "fumb" for *thumb*, "wabbit" for *rabbit*, or "tato" for *potato*). Research on typical speech development allows us to predict the ages at which each of these early types of articulation error should disappear and when mature production of certain sounds should be observed. For example, we would not expect to hear a 3-year-old child still saying "ba-ba" for *bottle*, although that same child is likely to still say "wabbit" for *rabbit*. Other speech errors, might involve reducing complex sound clusters such as /str/, /spl/, or /skr/ and are typical in child speech until 4 or 4.5 years (Lowe, 1994). Thus, many young children will say "*paghetti*," (spaghetti), "*paw-paw* " (Grandpa) or "*pash*" (splash). When a child continues to make specific articulation errors past the age when those errors should have disappeared, or if the child makes speech sound errors not observed in typical development, the child will require speech therapy to correct the problem.

The second major type of speech disorder that we see in young children is stuttering, which is classified as a *fluency disorder*, because it disrupts the smooth flow, or fluency, of the child's speech. Stuttering can take many different forms, and can range from mild to severe. Some children may repeat the first sound in a word ("t-t-t-talk"), the first syllable in a word ("pa-pa-pa-paper"), or the first word of a phrase ("my-my-my-my book"). Other children may prolong a sound or syllable ("baaaaaby"). Sometimes, this stuttering is paired with behaviors that suggest the child is really struggling with his speech. These behaviors may include eye blinking, facial grimaces, or tremors in the child's lips or jaw. Children who stutter may begin to avoid speaking situations or topics that require them to say certain words.

Just as it is typical for very young children to make certain types of articulation errors, it is also typical for young children to be dysfluent during the developmental period. Speech-language pathologists who work with speech disorders are able to evaluate the type and amount of a child's stuttering to determine if it is just normal, developmental nonfluency or if the child has a true fluency disorder. There have been great advances in the treatment of fluency disorders in recent years. Certainly, a child with serious dysfluencies should receive treatment. It can be a debilitating disorder for those who must live with it.

## The Importance of Early Identification of Language and Speech Disorders

We have noted that speech and language disorders affect only 10% of young children and that most such disorders are relatively mild. Given this information, the reader might wonder why we stress that it is so important for you to understand how language develops and to recognize the early signs of these disorders. The answer is simple: for that one child in 10 who has a true speech or language disorder, the impact is devastating! In Chapter 1 of this book, we discussed the central role that language plays in all of our lives and how language allows us to conduct the "business" of our everyday lives. For this reason, if not corrected early, even relatively minor problems can have serious consequences. This is especially true as children enter the world of formal education in first grade. Research has shown that children who have language disorders when they enter kindergarten will probably continue to have language problems in their later school years. What's more, these children are also likely to have problems with reading, spelling, and other school subjects as they get older (Catts, 1993; Fey, Catts, & Larrivee, 1995; Lockwood, 1994; Watkins, 1994).

Children with language disorders often fail to develop appropriate conversational skills as they get older (Brinton & Fujiki, 1989), and those with significant speech and language disorders are likely to avoid conversation altogether. Further, if the child's communication disorder makes it difficult or uncomfortable for others to have a conversation with the child, then classmates and even teachers may find themselves avoiding interaction with the child. This can be true for the child anywhere along the continuum of possible problems. Whether a child is nonverbal, has limited language facility, has severe articulation problems, or is a severe stutterer, he or she loses some part of his or her membership in the human social environment . Even when children have language disorders that seem relatively mild, research shows that they are likely to have fewer friends and to experience greater social rejection and isolation than children with normal language development (Rice, 1993).

Before the reader becomes too depressed about these unhappy consequences of childhood communication disorders, we should note again that current research is very encouraging about the benefits of early intervention for communication disorders. A recent review of intervention research involving young children with communication disorders summarized the findings of 56 studies published since 1987 (McLean & Cripe, 1997). The children in these studies were all younger than 6 years of age and had many different types of communication disorders, including unintelligible speech, stuttering, cleft palate, specific language impairments, and severe language delays. The results of these studies clearly demonstrated that early intervention for communication delays and disorders can be both effective and relatively efficient, if the disorder is identified and treated in early childhood.

We have seen that a variety of biological and environmental risk factors can affect the language development process and that about 10% of all children will have some type of communication delay or disorder resulting from one or more of these factors. We have also seen that these disorders can have harmful effects on children's future social and academic success. Finally, we have noted that many of these harmful effects can be reduced or avoided through early identification and treatment of communication disorders. For this reason, all professionals who come into daily contact with young children should have a basic understanding of how children develop their speech and language abilities. Even more important, professionals should be able to recognize the early signs of difficulty in the young child's learning of these critical skills and know what to do when they suspect a possible communication disorder. We hope that the information we have provided will allow you to identify children whose communication and language development seems to be delayed or disordered. In the remainder of this chapter, we discuss what you can do to support the language development of children with whom you interact and how you can help the child with a communication disorder.

## SUPPORTING LANGUAGE DEVELOPMENT FOR ALL CHILDREN

Professionals interact with young children in many different settings, including classrooms, day-care centers, doctor's offices, libraries, and playgrounds. In all of these settings, adults can support children's language development by remembering a few basic strategies. Not surprisingly, these strategies are based on the interaction patterns that characterize successful language development, which we discussed in some detail in Chapters 2, 3, and 4. These strategies are appropriate for supporting the language development of all young children, including those with and without disabilities that are beyond speech and language per se. By following these strategies, the professional will also create many opportunities to observe the child's developing communication and language skills and to identify children whose language seems to be delayed or disordered in some way. Let's briefly review these strategies:

1. **Listen to children's communication.** With very young children, or children with significant disabilities, we must remember to *listen with our eyes,* as well as with our ears. Try to *understand* what the child is communicating through gestures, facial expressions, words, and tone of voice. Let children know that you are interested in what they have to communicate by getting at their eye level and giving them your full attention when you are interacting with them. And remember to give the child a chance to communicate! Sometimes, as adults, it is hard for us to be quiet and wait for the child to take a turn in conversation. After you say something, *wait* for the child to respond.

2. **Respond to children's communication.** Perhaps the most important thing we can do to encourage children's communication development is to try to respond to the meaning and intent of the child's communication. By doing this, we reward the child's communication, and we also give the child feedback about the effectiveness and appropriateness of her or his communication act.

3. **Expand or emend children's communication.** It is often very natural and appropriate to incorporate children's words or gestures into our response; and to mod-

el a slightly more advanced way to express their meaning. For example, if a child points and says *"juice,"* you may respond by saying *"More* juice? Do you *want more* juice?" Of course, you must also *respond to the child's intent*—in this case, to get more juice. So, you would also want to give the child more juice, or explain why she can't have more juice right now. If you just expand and emend children's communication, without responding to their underlying intent, you will just frustrate the child!

4. **Encourage and reward children's communication.** Probably the most effective way to reward children's communication is by attending and responding in the ways we've already mentioned. You can also encourage children to communicate by making a comment about something they are doing and then *waiting* for them to respond or by asking an open-ended question and *waiting* for a response. Above all, let children know that you value communication and conversation and that you enjoy interacting with them. Remember that children can only learn how to communicate effectively, and how to use language appropriately, by engaging in lots of conversations. Silence is *not* golden!

5. **Provide opportunities to practice language in familiar interactive routines and games.** Research tells us that participating in predictable, *joint action routines* helps young children, including children with disabilities, develop competence as communication partners and language users (Ratner & Bruner, 1978; Snyder-McLean, Solomonson, McLean, & Sack, 1984). These routines begin with the very simple "peek-a-boo" and "gotcha" games that we play with infants. As children develop more skills in these interactive routines, we move to more elaborate games, like the make-believe tea parties in which toddlers love to engage their parents and grandparents ("Do you want more tea?"→"Yes Please") ("Do you want sugar"→"Yes—mmm this is good→Thank you!," "Do you want more tea?"→. . .)

As children become more skilled, they enjoy nursery rhymes and songs that create predictable routines, like "Old MacDonald Had a Farm" or "The Wheels on the Bus Go Round and Round." What all of these activities have in common is that they involve the child in a turn-taking interaction in which the child has a clear role and a predictable response. These familiar routines allow children to become competent social partners, and provide the context in which many new language skills are learned and practiced to perfection.

6. **Read to and with children.** Again, the research is clear: Children who have lots of experience with books become better language users and, of course, better readers. This experience begins with reading simple picture books to babies and toddlers. As young children become familiar with certain books, the book experience becomes one of *sharing*, and the child begins to "read" with the adult, filling in words or anticipating what will come on the next page. In fact, reading familiar books with children is a very effective example of the type of interactive routines we discussed earlier (Ratner, Parker, & Gardner, 1993). In addition to reading favorite and familiar books over and over again, it is also important to read some new books to children—books that are just a bit beyond their current language skills. These new books serve to introduce children to new words and new sentence forms and will soon become old familiar favorite books!

All of these strategies for interacting with children to promote their language development are consistent with current standards for "Developmentally Appropriate Practice" that have been identified by the National Association for the Education of Young Children (NAEYC). These standards for programs serving infants, toddlers, preschoolers, and young children are explained in detail in a manual produced by the NAEYC (Bredekamp & Copple, 1997).

## WHEN YOU SUSPECT A SPEECH OR LANGUAGE DISORDER

Professionals interacting with young children in environments that encourage communication and language, as described above, will occasionally notice a child who does not seem to be developing language at the same rate, or in the same ways, as other children of the same age. Although not all of these children actually have true language disorders, we know that 10% of young children do have language disorders of some type and that the earlier we can identify these children and provide appropriate services, the more effective our treatment will be. For this reason, a good rule of thumb is: When you suspect that a child may have a language disorder, it is better to refer the child for evaluation than to adopt a "wait and see" approach.

What should alert you to the possibility of a language disorder? Most basically, your understanding of the process and sequence of language development, described in the first six chapters of this book, is your best guide. If you notice that a child is not demonstrating the types of communication and language skills appropriate for his or her age, this is a "red flag" that the child *may* be showing the early signs of a language disorder. You can also compare the child's communication, speech, and language skills with those of other children with whom you interact who are the same age and from the same community. Finally, you may know that the child's background includes one or more of the risk factors identified earlier in this chapter. The presence of such risk factors, combined with an apparent delay or difference in the child's communication skills, increases the likelihood that you are seeing a true language disorder.

Another way in which we can identify children with possible language disorders is through a formal "screening" process. The term "screening" refers to a brief assessment that allows professionals to quickly identify children who *may* have some type of delay or disorder. In many Head Start and public school programs today, screenings for possible hearing, language and/or speech disorders are conducted with all preschool and elementary school-aged children. Most children who are Medicaid eligible are also eligible for a program of "Early and Periodic Screening, Diagnosis, and Treatment" (EPSDT) administered by the Medicaid agency in each state. This program provides periodic screening of children's health and developmental status and will support additional evaluations and treatment needed to address problems identified through these screenings. Also, Federal law requires that local education agencies provide free screenings for preschool children in their communities. Many school districts meet this requirement by scheduling one or more screening clinics each year. These clinics are widely advertised in local media. Other districts schedule individual screenings as young children are referred throughout the year.

Whether a child's possible language disorder is identified through a formal screening or through the types of informal observations discussed above, the next step remains the same: The child should be referred for a complete evaluation by a professional who specializes in communication disorders.

## Referring the Child for a Speech/Language/Hearing Evaluation

The first step in seeking a complete evaluation for any child is to discuss your concerns with the child's parent(s) or guardian. This is critical for several reasons. First, the law requires that the parent or guardian be informed about, and give permission for, this type of full-blown evaluation. Second, and more important, the parent(s) and other primary caregivers need to be involved in the evaluation if we are to get a complete and accurate picture of the child's language abilities and needs. Finally, if parents do not support and participate in the initial evaluation, they are less likely to understand and support any treatment recommendations that may result from that evaluation.

A comprehensive evaluation for a child with a suspected language disorder should begin with a hearing evaluation, conducted by an audiologist or speech-language pathologist, [3] to determine whether a hearing loss may be causing or contributing to the child's language difficulties. In addition, the comprehensive evaluation should include an in-depth assessment of the child's receptive and expressive language abilities. Depending on the child's level of development and the nature of the concerns about his or her language development, this evaluation may also include specific assessment of the child's nonverbal communication or speech articulation skills. This evaluation should be conducted by a qualified communication disorders specialist, with

[3] Audiologists and speech-language pathologists are certified by the American Speech-Language-Hearing Association. Most states today also require these professionals to be licensed to practice in their states.

input from the child's parent(s) and others who know the child well, including classroom personnel.

When this evaluation has been completed, the evaluator will provide a report to the parent(s) and the referring professional, if the parents have approved this. This report should include three major sections:

1. A *description* of the assessment process and results, including what instruments were administered and a summary of the child's performance in each area assessed;

2. A *determination*, based on these results, of whether the child does or does not have a communication disorder that requires treatment; and

3. A *recommendation* for the child's parents and school team. If the results indicate that the child does not have a communication disorder, then these recommendations will take the form of specific suggestions for parents and teachers to monitor and support the child's continued development, particularly in the area(s) of concern that led to the referral for evaluation. If the child is determined to have a communication disorder, then the recommendations should specify the type(s) of treatment and service that seem most appropriate for the child's needs.

## Intervention Services for Children With Communication Disorders

In the United States, most children with confirmed communication disorders will be eligible for services under the Federal "Individuals with Disabilities Education Act" (IDEA).[4] This law re-

[4] The IDEA was reauthorized by Congress in 1997, as Public Law 105–17. The U.S. Department of Education provides funding to each state to help subsidize the cost of these Federally mandated services. Services for families of infants and toddlers with disabilities (birth to age 3) are administered through a primary, lead agency designated by the Governor in each state. For children ages 3–21, these special services are administered through each state's Department of Education.

quires states to provide the types of comprehensive evaluation described above, at no cost to the child's family, for any child with a suspected disability. If that evaluation indicates that the child does have a disability and, therefore, needs some special education and/or related services to participate in the school curriculum, the IDEA also requires public schools to provide the needed services. Clearly, a disability affecting a child's language development will affect the child's ability to participate in all aspects of the school curriculum. Thus, services to address children's communication disorders will usually be provided through the IDEA, again at no cost to the child's parents.

For children younger than 3 years, Part C of the IDEA includes requirements for family centered "early intervention" services. These services may be provided through a number of different state and local service programs, and may be partially reimbursed through insurance or Medicaid/Medicare. Again, however, these services are provided at no cost to the child's family or on a sliding fee scale if state law requires this.

In addition to IDEA programs, a number of other state and local sources may provide needed intervention services for a child with a communication disorder. For example, Federal law requires that 10% of children enrolled in Head Start and Early Head Start programs be children with identified disabilities. Thus, these programs represent another community resource that can provide free services to children with communication disorders. Also, as noted earlier, the EPSDT program in each state will support needed speech/language therapy or audiology services for eligible children. Finally, for families who can afford (or who have insurance that will pay for) private therapy, these services can be obtained from speech-language therapists who work in private practices, or through a university-based speech and hearing clinic.

## Treatment for Communication Disorders

The nature and duration of treatment for a child's communication disorder will depend on the type of disorder the child has, as well as the severity of that disorder. In all cases, however, treatment should be based on a treatment plan that has been developed with the child's parent(s). If the child's intervention services are provided through IDEA, this treatment plan is called an "Individualized Educational Program" (IEP) or an "Individualized Family Service Plan" (IFSP) and may address additional needs of the child and family. At a minimum, any treatment plan for a communication disorder should include:

1. *One or more clearly stated goals or objectives.* What is the expected outcome of this treatment? What will the child be able to do as a result of this treatment? The expected outcome should be described in a way that can be observed or measured. This objective statement should also indicate an estimate of how long it will take to achieve this outcome.

2. *A plan for involving parents and other communication partners in the child's treatment.* Research tells us that early intervention for communication disorders is most effective when the child's communication partners understand and participate in the treatment. In many cases, especially with young children, treatment for the child's communication disorder will be integrated into ongoing daily activities in the child's home and classroom and will involve family members and classroom personnel directly in the treatment program. When the child's treatment is delivered in separate therapy sessions, this plan will take the form of suggestions for family members and other communication partners to help the child generalize, or "carry over" her new communication skill(s) into her daily interactions.

3. *A plan for measuring the child's progress.* A specific plan for monitoring the child's movement toward the expected outcome of treatment will allow the treatment team to make changes in the treatment plan, as needed. Parents or classroom personnel may be asked to participate in this monitoring process by providing reports on the child's use of targeted communication skills in everyday interactions.

### Treatment for Specific Speech and/or Language Disorders

The large majority of communication disorders in young children involve specific aspects of their speech or language production and may be described as mild to moderate in terms of severity. These include the types of articulation disorders, fluency disorders, and specific language impairments described earlier, in this chapter, as well as many cases of general language delay. Generally, treatment for these types of communication disorders is for a fixed period of time and the goal of treatment is complete remediation or elimination of the disorder.

For children with these disorders, effective treatment is likely to include a combination of "pull-out" therapy and treatment embedded into daily interactions in the child's home and classroom. In "pull-out" therapy, a communication disorders specialist will work with the child alone, or in a small group, to provide the child with intense instruction designed to correct specific speech or language errors. In these sessions, the therapist may use special techniques to help the child understand how to use the parts of his or her mouth and respiratory system to achieve correct sound production or carefully sequenced presentations of different grammatical constructions to help the child understand when to use different grammatical forms.

Generally, these intensive therapy sessions are short (an hour or less) and conducted only a few times a week. For this reason, it is very important for the child's parents and teachers to support and reinforce the child's therapy during the many hours and days when the child is not receiving therapy. For this purpose, the therapist will provide specific suggestions to the child's daily communication partners for ways to get the child to use her targeted speech or language skill in the context of her daily interactive routines at home and school (or daycare). The therapist should also provide these partners with guidelines for responding to the child's errors, as well as rewarding her correct productions.

### Treatment for Severe and Persistent Communication Disorders

As we noted earlier, a very small percentage of children will have severe communication disorders that cannot be remediated with short-term treatment. Such children may have speech that is completely unintelligible, or no speech at all; or they may have language that is limited to a few rote words or phrases, or no language at all. These disorders are typically associated with significant neurological impairment. In some cases, this impairment affects primarily the child's speech production and other fine motor abilities. In other cases, the child's communication disorder may be associated with a pervasive disorder that affects all aspects of the child's daily life. These associated disorders include autism, cerebral palsy, severe mental retardation, and traumatic brain injury.

For these children, the goal of intervention is to improve the quality and effectiveness of their communication and, thus, the quality of their lives. It is not expected that treatment will "cure" the child's communication disorder; and it is likely that treatment services will be needed throughout the child's school years and, in many cases, throughout life. Nonetheless, for children with these severe, multiple disabilities, communication is the skill area that is often given the highest priority for treatment by the child's family and intervention team. This is because parents and teachers, alike, recognize that the ability to communicate with other people is essential for the child's successful participation in school, work, and social activities.

Intervention services for children with severe, multiple disabilities are provided by an interdisciplinary team of professionals with special expertise related to the child's specific disabilities. Thus, the full treatment team for a child with complex and multiple disabilities may include a physical therapist, an occupational therapist, a pediatric neurologist, a psychologist, an audiologist, a speech-language pathologist, an assistive technology specialist, and/or a special education teacher. This team will work closely with the child's family and classroom personnel to plan and implement the child's intervention program.

Intervention typically includes two types of activities: (a) treatment activities designed to help the child acquire new skills, or improve skills she already has and (b) program supports and accommodations that will allow the child to participate most effectively in daily activities and interactions. Treatment activities to help the child master new communication skills will usually be integrated throughout the child's day; and all personnel who interact regularly with the child will be involved in helping the child learn to use these skills. Needed accommodations for children with severe disabilities may include training family members and school personnel to recognize and understand the child's nonverbal communication or providing appropriate assistive technology[5] to allow the child to communicate, and perform daily activities more independently. For children with severe communication disorders, the most commonly needed type of assistive technology is an "alternative/augmentative communication" (AAC) system. This is usually some type of board with a display of pictures, symbols, letters, and/or words that the child indicates when she or he wants to communicate. These boards range from very simple boards, containing a few pictures of favorite things, to highly sophisticated, microcomputer systems that produce fluent synthetic speech as the user enters letters and words. Young children with severe disabilities may progress through several of these AAC systems as their language abilities develop. For other children, particularly children who are deaf, the AAC system used may be a formal sign language.[6] Regardless of the AAC system selected for a child, all of the child's daily communication partners need to receive adequate support and training in the use of that system so that they can interact effectively with the child.

## WHEN YOU HAVE A CHILD WITH AN IDENTIFIED COMMUNICATION DISORDER IN YOUR SETTING

There is a growing recognition today that children with disabilities, including communication disabilities, need to be included in programs and activities with their typically developing peers. Children with disabilities learn by watching and interacting with

---

[5] Assistive technology refers to any device that is used to increase, maintain, or improve the functional capabilities of a child with disabilities and any services related to those devices. Assistive technology includes such things as wheelchairs, communication boards, hearing aids, computer software that reads screen text aloud, etc. The IDEA requires schools to consider and provide, as needed, appropriate assistive technology for any child with a disability.

[6] There are a number of different sign languages. The language used by adults in America's "deaf culture" is American Sign Language (ASL). ASL has its own morphology and syntax and is valued by deaf adults as a very efficient and effective means of communication. For school-aged children, another commonly used sign language is "Signing Exact English," or SEE. SEE consists of signs that correspond to standard English morphemes and signed utterances or sentences conform to standard English syntax.

other children, and they benefit from the high expectations that we have for all children in these settings. We have found that even children with the most severe disabilities can flourish when they are allowed to participate in normal daycare, preschool, community, and school environments. In such settings, we have seen children with severe disabilities develop more skills and become more independent than we ever thought possible. Further, the Federal courts have repeatedly ruled that policies calling for the segregation of children with disabilities into separate classes and schools is a violation of their civil rights. In addition, the Americans with Disabilities Act requires that community programs and retail services, as well as public schools, must provide any reasonable accommodations needed to allow the participation of children with disabilities.

For all of these reasons, there is a growing trend toward greater inclusion of children with disabilities in typical community recreation, day-care, preschool, and public school programs. This means that professionals working in these settings today are likely to be interacting—perhaps for the first time—with children who have a variety of disabilities, including communication disorders. If you are one of these professionals, there are a number of things you can do to support the child with a communication disorder in your setting.

The first thing to remember is: Trust yourself! Children with disabilities are children first; and they are more like other children their age than different. The experience and knowledge you have about interacting with children, and about your program or setting, are your most important guides for including a child with disabilities in your program. You do not need to be a disability or communication disorders specialist; just be yourself and let the child be a child. Beyond this general rule of thumb, here are a few other points to keep in mind:

1. The same strategies we discussed earlier for supporting the language development of all children are also appropriate for children with communication disorders. Listening and responding to the child's communication; expanding, emending, and encouraging communication; providing familiar interactive routines; and reading with the child are especially important for the child with a communication disorder.

2. Include the child in all group activities and interactions. Let the child know that you expect him or her to communicate and participate! If you are not sure how the child can be appropriately included in some activities, ask her communication disorders specialist for suggestions.

3. Ask about the child's IEP or IFSP, if you were not involved when it was developed. This will tell you the child's current communication goals, and what services the child is receiving. Also ask the child's parents and support personnel about any specific strategies that they use to support the child's communication.

4. If you are the child's teacher, you should be a member of her IEP or IFSP planning team. Even if you are not a member of this team, it is important for you to communicate your observations, concerns, and successes with this child to the child's parents and support personnel so that they can share this information with the team and, if appropriate, respond to your concerns.

5. If you are working with a child who has severe disabilities, get to know the different specialists who work with the child and let them know if you have questions or concerns about the child's communication. If the child is using an AAC system, make sure that someone on the team provides you (and others in your setting) with whatever training or support you need to be able to interact with the child using this system.

## CONCLUSIONS

Professionals working with young children must understand *how* children learn language. They also need to know *why* children learn language, and *what* it is that they learn as they progress from their first attempts at words at about 1 year of age to the thousands of well-structured sentences that they can produce at about 3 years of age. It is our hope that this book has helped you to develop this understanding and has given you confidence in your ability to play a critical supporting role in the language development of *all* the children with whom you interact every day.

## SUMMARY

- Problems with speech and language development affect about 10% of all preschool children.

- Intervention can be very effective in treating these disorders, especially if they are identified early.

- Educators and other professionals who work with young children can support language development in all children by employing strategies that are based on the interaction patterns that characterize successful language development.

- The same professionals can play a critical role in helping to identify children who may have a communication disorder and referring them for appropriate evaluation and needed services.

- Teachers, day-care providers, and other professionals can work with a child's intervention team to support the treatment plan for any child in their setting who has an identified communication disorder.

### References

American Speech-Language-Hearing Association. (1993). Definitions of communication disorders and variations. *Asha, 35*(Suppl. 10), 40–41.

American Speech-Language-Hearing Association, Joint Subcommittee of the Executive Board on English Language Proficiency. (1998). Students and professionals who speak English with accents and non-standard dialects: Issues and recommendations. Position statement and technical report. *Asha, 40*(Suppl. 18), 28–31.

Bredekamp, S., & Copple, C. (Eds.). (1997). *Developmentally appropriate practice in early childhood programs* (rev. ed.). Washington, DC: National Association for the Education of Young Children.

Brinton, B., & Fujiki, M. (1989). *Conversational management with language-impaired children*. Rockville, MD: Aspen Press.

Catts, H. W. (1993). The relationship between speech-language impairments and reading disabilities. *Journal of Speech and Hearing Research, 36*, 948–958.

Fey, M. E., Catts, H. W., & Larrivee, L. S. (1995). Preparing preschoolers for the academic and social challenges of school. In M. E. Fey, J. Windsor, & S. F. Warren (Eds.), *Language intervention: Preschool through the elementary years* (pp. 3–38). Baltimore: Paul H. Brookes.

Hart, B., & Risley, T. R. (1995). *Meaningful differences in the everyday experience of young American children.* Baltimore: Paul H. Brookes.

Lockwood, S. L. (1994). Early speech and language indicators for later learning problems: Recognizing a language organization disorder. *Infants and Young Children, 7*(2), 43–52.

Lowe, R. J. (1994). *Phonology: Assessment and intervention applications in speech pathology.* Baltimore: Williams & Wilkins.

McLean, J. E., McLean, L. K. S., Brady, N. C., & Etter, R. (1991). Communication profiles of two types of gesture using nonverbal persons with severe to profound mental retardation. *Journal of Speech and Hearing Research, 34,* 294–308.

McLean, L. K., & Cripe, J. W. (1997). The effectiveness of early intervention for children with communication disorders. In M. J. Guralnick (Ed.), *The effectiveness of early intervention* (pp. 349–428). Baltimore: Paul H. Brookes.

Office of Scientific and Health Reports. (1988). *Developmental speech and language disorders: Hope through research* (NIH Publication Pamphlet 88–2757). Bethesda, MD: National Institute of Neurological and Communicative Disorders and Stroke.

Ratner, N., & Bruner, J. (1978). Games, social exchange, and the acquisition of language. *Journal of Child Language, 5,* 391–401.

Rice, M. L. (1993). "Don't talk to him: He's Weird": The role of language in early social interactions. In A. P. Kaiser & D. B. Gray (Eds.), *Enhancing children's communication: Research foundations for intervention* (pp. 139–158). Baltimore: Paul H. Brookes.

Samaroff, A. J. (1975). Early influence on development: Fact or fancy? *Merrill-Palmer Quarterly, 21,* 267–294.

Snyder-McLean, L., Solomonson, B., McLean, J., & Sack, S. (1984). Structuring joint action routines: A strategy for facilitating communication and language development in the classroom. *Seminars in Speech and Language, 5,* 213–228.

Watkins, R. V. (1994). Specific language impairments in children: An introduction. In R. V. Watkins & M. L. Rice (Eds.), *Specific language impairments in children* (pp. 1–16). Baltimore: Paul H. Brookes.

# INDEX